I0440278

Decoding Myth Information

A Treatise
on the Regulation of
Herbal Medicine in the UK

Decoding Myth Information

A Treatise
on the Regulation of
Herbal Medicine in the UK

By
Robert Scott

Copyright © 2010 Robert Scott

ISBN 9878-1-4452-7927-5

All rights reserved. Apart from any fair dealing for the purpose of private study, research, criticism or review, as permitted under the Copyright, Designs and Patent Act 1988.

Disclaimer:

While every effort has been made to provide accurate information, the author and publishers do not assume and hereby disclaim any liability to any party for loss or damage caused by errors in this report.

~ DEDICATION ~

To All Herbalists Who in the spirit of Nicholas Culpepper
have practised and protected the traditional practice and
philosophy of natural medicine in the face of adversity
throughout the ages.

Contents

Foreword

"I speak the truth not as much as I would, but as much as I dare and I dare a little more as I grow older." (Montague)

Freedom to choose the appropriate healthcare for one's self and family is an unalienable, natural human right. For the people of Britain this freedom has been enshrined in a Royal Charter since the reign of King Henry the VIII.

The Royal Charter, also known as the 'Herbalist Charter' provides a secure foundation for people to choose health care in accordance with their beliefs and values, which is safe, effective and natural. Similarly healers and practitioners have also been able to care and serve people for over 450 years under the protection of this Royal Charter.

However since this Charter, various groups, based on narrow self interests and greed, have attempted to stop this choice, by creating fears of various kinds.

This latest fear against herbal medicines and herbalists is the 'Trojan horse' tactic used by a few elitist herbalists. They are using the twin smoke screens of 'public safety' and 'European legislation' to convey false messages and are endangering the British peoples' freedom to practice and benefit from herbal medicine.

It is ironic that when natural therapies and wisdom based on traditions of health and well being are having a renaissance across the world, British people are in danger of losing one of their long cherished rights, the freedom to choose herbal products and consult herbalists.

Robert Scott's well researched work: 'DECODING MYTH–INFORMATION', comes at a time when 'spin doctors' are spreading webs of deceit and misinformation about the future of herbalists and herbal medicine in Britain.

Robert Scott's book is necessary reading for those who wish to maintain the peoples' freedom to practice and benefit from herbal medicine and the experience of herbalists that have been safely practising for the last 450 years under the Royal Charter of Henry VIII.

Hakim M. Salim Khan
M.D. (M.A.) M.H. F.G.N.I. (England) D.O. (London)

Acknowledgements

The preparation of this treatise would not have been possible without the editorial and personal support of my beloved wife Marilyn.

I would also like to thank the past and present members of the National Institute of Herbal Medicine, the past and present members the Unified Register of Herbal Practitioners and the past and present members of the International Register of Consultant Herbalists and Homoeopaths for the current and historical detail that has been necessary to develop the balanced perspective, offered in this treatise.

I would further like to thank Mr Mohammed Salim Kahn, for initially suggesting that I compile the past few years' correspondence and research within a single document.

It is my hope that in uniting many scattered fragments of information, the world of Herbal Medicine, in all its diverse traditions, will become better informed and more confident facing the challenges of the 21st century. At the same time I hope we can maintain the insight, philosophy and cultural heritage that has been handed down to us faithfully by generations past.

Please note that direct quotes from other source material will appear in **_bold italic_** text.

***

Introduction

In recent years there has been an ever increasing pressure from the EU to regulate Herbal Medicine. This gave rise to concerns about the continued right to practice, historically enjoyed by Herbalists under a Royal Charter issued by Henry VIII (see appendix).

There had already been a divergence between two schools of thought within Herbal Medicine. Whereas one branch maintained the traditional philosophy and practice, the other group pursued another direction more centred on biochemistry and reductionist science. Under growing concern for their future, the modernist branch of herbal medicine has championed the cause of the most challenging level of regulation to secure their future.

To this end, its training was given over to the university system, and in the process out of the hands of experienced herbal practitioners. Although the university system has been able to confer graduate status on those it has trained, it has come at the cost of reducing the traditional craft to an academic science.

This abandonment of the traditional aspects of Herbal Medicine has now become increasingly unpopular, and has led to the closure of several university courses, through lack of support. In an attempt to counter this, prospective students have been led to believe that if they do not undertake "modernist" approved training, qualifications achieved through traditional training might not be recognized in the future.

The uncertainty that this has produced could seriously threaten the future availability of genuine traditional Herbal Medicine and its practitioners.

In attempt to create and maintain its claim that only modernist trained Herbalists would be able to continue to practice; and to protect its own position in the process, its champions have put forward a raft of misinformation to protect their failing agenda.

The need to bring some clarity to dispel the confusion has become increasingly apparent. This gives rise to the question about how this might be achieved.

When it was first suggested that I put together the treatise on the subject of the regulation of Herbal Medicine, I was confronted with the question of where to start.

For reasons described above, it was immediately apparent that this would have to be the consideration of the quintessential nature of Herbal Medicine, as without this, the subject of its regulation would be devoid of meaning. Despite this, it was stated:-

"The Working Group did not consider the details of individual professional groups as part of their work." [1]

This could be seen as the first official indication that any proposals would be fundamentally incompatible with the nature and philosophy of individual professional groups. The imposition of regulation under such circumstances would therefore necessitate an enforced alteration to the philosophy and practice of the profession, to fit in with the requirements of regulation.

Here it should be noted that on the Health Professionals' Council (HPC) website it is stated that one of the alleged benefits of regulation is the protection of the traditions.

This is the first of many paradoxical anomalies, contradictions and non-sequiturs that will be addressed in this treatise.

It will also be noted that during this treatise, the same documentation may be quoted on several occasions to demonstrate a number of anomalous statements that had been made on the subject of regulation.

***

---

[1] Report from the Working Group on Extending Professional Regulation 2009 (page 7)

1

The Concept of Regulation

In the light of the considerable degree of confusion that has been put forward on this subject, it is necessary to investigate exactly what the concept of the regulation of Herbal Medicine entails.

One way or another, regulation of Herbal Medicine relates to three individual areas of interest.

1) The use of the "title" Herbalist in relation to the various traditions.

2) The "practice" or area of activity of the Herbalist.

3) The "medicine" or substances used by the practitioner.

These three specific and individual areas have been discussed at great length within the Steering Group Report[2] and the subsequent Interim and Final Reports from the Working Group on Extending Regulation (WG on EPR)[3] as well as in the document "COM(2008) 584 final (the) COMMUNICATION FROM THE COMMISSION TO THE COUNCIL AND THE EUROPEAN PARLIAMENT concerning the Report on 2a of Directive 2001/83/EC, as amended by Directive 2004/24/EC, on specific

---

[2] Report to Ministers from The Department of Health Steering Group on the Statutory Regulation of Practitioners of Acupuncture, Herbal Medicine, Traditional Chinese Medicine and Other Traditional Medicine Systems Practised in the UK May 2008

[3] Extending Professional Regulation Working Group *Interim Report: Protecting the public by ensuring that workforce standards are met*(6.6.2008) and *The Report of the Working Group on Extending Professional Regulation* (16.6.2009)

provisions applicable to traditional herbal medicinal products (Document on the basis of Article 16i of Directive 2001/83/EC)."

Protected Title

The use of "protected title" relates to who is, or is not, able to describe themselves (in this case) as either an "Herbalist" or "Acupuncturist". Up until now the only definition of Herbalist was the one laid down in King Henry VIII's Royal Charter. This is particularly important as it has been proposed that the regulation of Herbal Medicine, Acupuncture and Traditional Chinese Medicine (TCM) should be the control of the use of "protected title".

This is discussed at length in the chapter "Models of Regulation".

As the models of regulation controlling the use of "title" do not cover the area of activity per se, an individual would remain free to undertake the activities associated with the practice of Herbal Medicine, without being regulated, as long as he does not call himself a Herbalist. A similar situation is already the case with Osteopaths, in which unregulated therapists practice under an unprotected title.

The group recognised that there is a wide range of titles in use by these practitioners, and that not all of these titles could be protected.[4]

This demonstrates that regulation by protected title is little more than an expensive exercise in semantics. It does not protect the tradition; it does not protect the public and would only seem to benefit the regulatory "industry" that is paid to administer it.

Regulated Practice

The option of regulating the "practice" rather than the "title" was also discussed within the Steering Group Report and subsequent reports from the WG on EPR. This is also discussed in the chapter headed "Models of

---

[4] Steering Group Report (page 15)

Regulation". Any move to adopt the regulation of "practice" would inevitably give rise to a catalogue of unintended consequences.

It is already the case that Acupuncture is practised by doctors and nurses within the NHS, without being fully qualified within the profession. In the event of regulation by "protected title" it has been proposed that this practice should be allowed to continue, as long as the unqualified user of Acupuncture does not call himself (or herself) an Acupuncturist.

"The proposals highlighted in the Pittilo report stated the statutory regulated profession, e.g. doctor or nurse, would still have to meet the standards of acupuncture, herbal medicine or TCM set by the primary regulator (i.e. the HPC or some other regulatory body)."[5]

The WG on EPR report does go on to discuss the practicalities involved in extending a network of cross referenced arrangements, whereby therapists in one regulated therapy might practice another regulated therapy by similar arrangements.

This would have by-passed the need to pay multiple regulation annual fees, but was considered too complicated and expensive to administer. The message here is clearly "if it is too expensive for Government to fund, let the therapist pay, and pass the cost onto the patient."

This strategy is euphemistically termed "self financing".

One of the main planks of the official argument that has been put forward for the Statutory Regulation of Herbal Medicine, Acupuncture and Traditional Chinese Medicine, has been the alleged danger that these therapies present to the public. It is therefore difficult to support the point of view that a partially trained Acupuncturist poses less of a risk than a fully trained one.

A nurse or a doctor may already be statutory regulated in their own professions, but the practice of Acupuncture is a separate discipline

---

[5] Sharon Corner European & Specialist Legislation Team, Workforce Directorate, Department of Health (26.6.2009)

altogether, and a standard of achieved excellence in one does not automatically confer excellence of expertise in another.

If it is the therapist that needs to be regulated, this could be achieved by a licensing scheme independent of the therapy itself, and would prevent the necessity for multiple regulation fees for a practitioner undertaking more than one (otherwise regulated) therapy.

This point again highlights the difference between the regulation of "title" (the therapist) and the regulation of "practice" (the therapy) and the sort of anomalous situations that the proposed regulation might give rise to.

The control of herbal medicine products come under the auspices of the Herbal Medicines Product Directive (THMPD). This has nothing whatever to do with the regulation of the practitioner. It is evident that there has been a high degree of confusion about the nature of these concepts. Although rumours have been perpetuated to the contrary, the regulation of the practitioner by the Health Professionals' Council does not entail the admittance of the regulated therapist into the NHS.

Regulation only denotes control, and not acceptance. It is already the case that therapy only has to be "approved" by a local health authority for it to be used and paid for by the NHS (as is already the case with Acupuncture). Any argument to the contrary, is not only unsupported by the facts, but would also constitute an attempt to mislead the unwary practitioner into accepting a totally inappropriate level of regulation.

"If a practitioner is regulated by statute, it does not necessarily mean their services are available on the NHS; this is currently the case with many chiropractors and osteopaths. It would be a matter for local commissioners to decide whether to fund CAM therapies on the NHS. Indeed many CAM therapists choose to only practise privately"[6]

---

[6] Sharon Corner (European and Specialist Legislation Team, Workforce Directorate, Department Of Health, 26th of June 2009.

Licensed Herbal Products

The approval and licensing of herbal medicine products does not denote the acceptance or approval of the tradition with which it is associated. This further confirms that the therapist and the materials used, in the conduct of the therapy, are totally separate issues. The general argument to support the concept of licensing herbal medicine products, has, in part, been built on the idea that this would prevent products (generally relating to either TCM or Ayurvedic medicine) contaminated with toxic heavy metals from being marketed, despite the fact that Mercury, a toxic heavy metal with well-known adverse side-effects, is being widely used in allopathic medicine.

It has however been pointed out that such inclusions are already illegal. It is also already illegal to make unsubstantiated claims of "benefit", relating to a product.[7]

As the inclusion of toxic heavy metals is already illegal, the failure is clearly demonstrated as being the lack of enforcement of the current regulations. This in turn demonstrates that the remedy to the situation is the enforcement of existing legislation, not the creation of yet another tier of legal instruments.

"On the other hand, it should be emphasised that Community legislation on medicinal products, in particular Directive 2001/83/EC laying down the procedures for placing products on the market, follows a product-specific approach and does not attempt to provide a framework for the regulation of traditions of medical practice".............. "the set of requirements a simplified registration procedure under Directive 2004/24/EC is not appropriate for a global regulation of such medicinal practices. The regulation of such

---

[7] Document 3 paragraph 18 "Briefing Paper from Michael McIntyre, Chair of the European Herbal and Traditional Medicine Practitioners Association on the Statutory Regulation of Practitioners of Acupuncture, Herbal Medicine, Traditional Chinese Medicine and Other Traditional Medicine Systems Practised in the UK" (previously available on the EHTPA website).

additions would demand different approach from that introduced by directive 2004/24/EC."[8]

The alleged purpose of regulation is the protection of the public, and not the professional advancement of the therapist.

"In the past there has been a danger that the extension of professional regulation to new groups has been overly driven by the aspirations of emerging professional groups themselves, as a means to establish themselves as safe and effective players in the health care arena.

This has at times led to the use of the terminology of "aspirant" groups. This term was introduced by the HPC for the purpose of indicating when applications for regulation were made to it by groups who were seeking recognition as "professions".

The term has since become associated with those groups seeking regulation through emphasising the risks inherent in their professions in order to secure their positions within health care, for reasons of status and market position as well as for reasons of public protection and patient safety.

The Working Group agreed that continuing this approach to Statutory Regulation would not only have significant costs to the public purse and to the bureaucracy associated with spiralling legislation but would sustain an approach that did not have protection of the public as its primary concern: regulation is there primarily to serve the public, not the professions, and consideration of extension of regulation needs to start from the perspective of risk to the public and consider from that

---

[8] COM(2008) 584 final (the) "COMMUNICATION FROM THE COMMISSION TO THE COUNCIL AND THE EUROPEAN PARLIAMENT concerning the Report on 2a of Directive 2001/83/EC, as amended by Directive 2004/24/EC, on specific provisions applicable traditional herbal medicinal products (Document on the basis of Article 16i of Directive 2001/83/EC)." (page 10)

perspective which professional groups should be drawn into the system and how best to do so." [9]

Unfortunately exactly the opposite motivation might be implied in the Steering Group Report by the inference that the HPC regulation might be used as a marketing device.

The HPC already offers an 'e-kit' for registrants with images that can be downloaded for use in advertising material encouraging said users to reinforce their registration with a logo. It also offers other public facing material for registered professionals to use, including leaflets, posters and window-stickers. [10]

There has been a further widely held belief that a statutory regulated practitioner would have access to unlicensed manufactured herbal medicine products, when otherwise this would not be the case.

This subject will be dealt with later in the chapter "The Benefits of Statutory Regulation Fact or Myth".

Ever since the time of Nicolas Culpepper, and even before that, Herbalists have had to fight to maintain independence from the influence and control of the pharmacists and the practitioners of allopathic medicine.

Proposals for the more onerous forms of regulation would place Herbal Medicine squarely into their area of domination. In the light of the change of relationship between patient and therapist that is inherent in the concept of regulation, it would constitute the triumph of fear over trust. This could only be to the detriment of the healing relationship, as well as the healing that flows from it.

Further to this, is the totally false premise that laws, rules and regulations actually have a significant effect in changing or controlling the behaviour of the regulated individual.

---

[9] WG on EPR report, page 43

[10] Steering Group Report (page 16)

This is amply demonstrated by the mere fact that Her Majesty's Prisons are so overcrowded that the judiciary have been issued guidelines to avoid issuing sentences of incarceration wherever possible.

Had the existence of laws, rules and regulations actually been an effective deterrent to criminal activity, none would have been committed, and so there would be no necessity to provide establishments of captivity and correction in the first place.

In addition to this, it is the excess of regulation, by virtue of its own self inflicted complexity, that inevitably paralyses the regulated area of activity and prevents it fulfilling its purpose.

***

2

History

As Herbal Medicine yet again faces the unsought challenges of a changing world, it is important for Herbalists to remember their heritage and those aspects of it which they need to protect as they move forward into the future. Conformity can only come at the expense of the extraordinary. It would be a tragedy if a level of excellence, standing at the pinnacle of millennia of empirical experience, were to be cast aside to fit the current fashion of limited reductionist science.

In order to create a unified voice to represent the interests of Herbal Medicine, in all its diverse traditions, an organisation was formed in 1993, which is now known as the European Herbal Traditional Practitioners Association (EHTPA).

This is a small group comprised of representatives drawn from Professional Associations (PAs), the Registers of the various traditions.

Ayurveda
Ayurvedic Practitioners Association

Chinese Herbal Medicine/Traditional Chinese Medicine
Register of Chinese Herbal Medicine

Traditional Tibetan Medicine
British Association of Traditional Tibetan Medicine

Western Herbal Medicine
Association of Master Herbalists
College of Practitioners of Phytotherapy

National Institute of Medical Herbalists
Unified Register of Herbal Practitioners

EHTPA Associate Members
National Herbalists (Ireland)
Kommitten för Alternativ Medicin (Committee for Alternative Medicine), Sweden[11]

NB. The International Register of Consultant Herbalists and Homoeopaths (IRCH) was a member of the EHTPA until its resignation on the 5th June 2009. Significantly, the IRCH was formerly entered in the "Western Herbal Medicine" section.

The EHTPA Council is made up of representatives from each member Professional Association. These are as follows:-

Tony Booker	Jane Gray
David Broom	Sascha Kriese
Alison Lunnell	Vicki Pitman
Peter Conway	Peter Jackson-Maine
Geoffrey Mead	Brion Sweeney
Elizabeth Lyden	Jay Mackinnon

Michael McIntyre	**Chair EHTPA**
Peter Eaton	**Secretary**
Lynn Copcutt	**Chair Accreditation Board**
Phillip Lockett	**Chair, Education Board**[12]

Although this list has been copied from the EHTPA website (where this information is already in the public domain) on the 25th of November 2009,

---

[11] This information is publicly available on the EHTPA website

[12] This information (as verified 16.12.2009) is publicly available on the EHTPA website

Mr David Broom (MIRCH) resigned from this organisation in January 2009, and so even this list overstates the size of its membership.

Historically these professional associations have set and maintained the standards of their membership through Voluntary Self-Regulation (VSR). This system of regulation was controlled by the experts in the individual areas of practice, and has served the public well since its inception.

It has always been an integral part of every individual constitution that the highest professional standards should be maintained, and any behaviour bringing the profession into disrepute would bring about the deregulation of the guilty party.

In spite of the established success of Voluntary Self-Regulation, changes to the tried and tested formula were put forward to allegedly "save" the future of Herbal Medicine.

It is however interesting that one of the arguments put forward for Statutory Regulation of Acupuncture, Herbal/Traditional Medicine and TCM, was not entirely based on the alleged dangers of these therapies, but the fear that the public might favour them and reject allopathic treatment.

"Their Lordships made this recommendation because, as they explained, "these therapies carry inherent risk, beyond the intrinsic risk that all CAMs (Complementary and Alternative Medicine Systems) pose, which is the omission of conventional medical treatment." [13]

This calls into question the Government's commitment to the concept of choice. A comparison of the inherent dangers of allopathic medicine was not undertaken. This will be covered in a later chapter.

Under the threat of the reported impending changes in legislation, relating to the authority of traditional practitioners to make their own diagnosis, an alternative system called Statutory Self Regulation (SSR) was proposed. Strictly speaking, this change of authority would have been largely irrelevant

---

[13] House of Lords Select Committee on Science and Technology (Section 5.53)

to the traditional practitioner. The traditional therapist diagnoses the patient, not the illness, and offers treatment on that basis.

This is the systems approach, which acknowledges the multiplicity of routes to illness which need to be treated according to their nature, as opposed to the symptoms approach of modern medical practice, which fails to differentiate between different individuals presenting the same outward symptoms.

Although the practitioner of allopathic medicine "diagnoses", the practitioner of traditional medicine "evaluates".

At least one of the EHTPA Professional Associations, the International Register of Consultant Herbalists and Homoeopaths (IRCH) was persuaded to set aside their concerns over the change of regulatory basis, and follow that path of SSR. The members of the IRCH were told that by adopting Statutory Self Regulation, they would improve their professional status and promote the use of Herbal Medicine within the NHS.

The claim that regulation would give the practitioner access to work within the NHS was however entirely misleading. The IRCH membership was however also warned:-

"SSR puts herbal medicine into the State arena, in which conventional medical discourse prevails, and it leaves by definition to some interference by Government, since statutory regulated health professions have appointments made on to their governing councils by the Secretary of State".[14]

This highlighted the conflict between the basic philosophies of traditional Herbal Medicine and mainstream allopathic practice, and indicates a fundamental incompatibility of approach. It should be noted that even at this stage, confusion was being introduced between Statutory Self-Regulation (SSR) and Statutory Regulation (SR). This confusion has been carried forward into more recent times, and even challenges the validity of the

---

[14] Article by Nick Lampert, April 2001 published in The Journal of Natural Medicine, Volume V Issue 4 Winter/Spring 2001/2

Steering Group Report, and all the other reports that it subsequently gave rise to.

At the time when the EHTPA Chairman sat as a stakeholder chair of the Steering Group Committee, the National Institute of Medical Herbalists (NIMH) was still democratically bound to the pursuit of Statutory Self-Regulation. NIMH is by far the largest Professional Association in the practice of Western Herbal Medicine in the EHTPA. The vote to change its policy from SSR to SR did not occur until November 2008, with only 28% of the membership in favour.

The vast majority of the membership either felt insufficiently informed of the issues involved in this change or actually voted against it. Active debate on the subject of the pros and cons of Statutory Regulation was inhibited by the closing down of the NIMH members' forum soon after comments doubting the future viability of Statutory Regulation were posted upon it.

The imposition of a motion approved by only 28% of the membership has led to resignations from the membership of NIMH. This in turn has resulted in an increase in the number of experienced and reputable Herbalists who are now working outside the existing structure of Voluntary Self-Regulation.

These former NIMH members are now serving the public under the traditional arrangements described as "caveat emptor" (buyer beware) which will be discussed in a later chapter.

Therefore, from the point of view of regulation, the attempt to impose Statutory Regulation has been entirely counter-productive.

The members of another EHTPA Professional Association, The International Register of Consultant Herbalists and Homoeopaths (IRCH) were never even offered a vote on this crucial change. The IRCH subsequently resigned from the EHTPA, as it saw that the change in policy was not in line with its own philosophy, and recognized it to be contrary to the interests of Traditional Herbal Medicine in general.

According to the stated policy of a fourth EHTPA Professional Association, the Master Herbalists that there should be:-

"A herbalist in every home, a practitioner in every town"
Dr John Christopher (1909 – 1983)

Every home should have a table to eat round and home cooked food upon it; every home should have a herbal medicine cupboard.
Barbara Griggs

It is more important to know what sort of person has a disease than to know what sort of disease a person has.
Hippocrates".

Such a doctrine is incompatible with the idea that traditional practice of Herbal Medicine should be restricted to state regulated practitioners only. As a result of these circumstances, a democratic mandate had never been established to change the EHTPA approved policy on the proposals for the future regulation of Western Herbal Medicine.

The mandate for SR was only sought five months after the publication of the Steering Group Report in May 2008. Even then, such support as it did receive clearly did not reflect the informed opinion of the majority of practitioners. The question of mandate becomes important, because the EHTPA Chairman himself stressed the importance of his own influence on the Steering Group Committee on which he was a stakeholder member.[15] This circumstance is of particular importance on two counts.

1) It undermines the validity of both the Steering Group Report and any subsequent reports based upon it.

2) It invalidates the subsequent application for Statutory Regulation.

Here it should be pointed out that the previously adopted option of Statutory Self Regulation was not even included in the report from the WG

---

[15]EHTPA Briefing paper dated 7.5.2008, previously available on the EHTPA website from the EHTPA [15] Extracts quoted from the Master Herbalists website homepage.

on EPR, and Statutory Regulation must be applied for, and cannot be imposed unless a considerable danger has been established to justify it.

"....the suitability of non-statutory forms of regulation should have been considered and there should be a compelling argument for transferring any existing system of non-Statutory Regulation to a statutory system."[16]

This was a crucial statement, as it had already been stated in the House of Lords Select Committee on Science and Technology Report that Herbal Medicine, Acupuncture and Traditional Chinese Medicine *"already had a coherent voluntary regulation system and a credible, if incomplete evidence base."*

The juxtaposition of these two statements would appear to indicate that any attempt to impose Statutory Regulation would be unconstitutional.

The Chairman of the EHTPA wrote to Mr Ben Bradshaw MP, who was then a Minister at the Department of Health, indicating a much wider support for the Statutory Regulation of Herbal Medicine than can actually be substantiated, because, even at that time, the membership of all the qualifying professional associations had not voted on this subject.[17]

It was only after this, that the recommendation supporting the Statutory Regulation of Herbal Medicine, Acupuncture and Traditional Chinese Medicine was issued by the Registrar of the Health Professionals' Council (HPC). The recommendation was dated 5th of November 2008.[18] As has been indicated above, at the time the recommendation for the Statutory Regulation of Herbal Medicine was made to the Secretary of State for Health (then Mr Allen Johnson MP) there was no majority mandate for this amongst practitioners of Western Herbal Medicine.

---

[16] WG on EPR Interim Report (page 26)

[17] EHTPA briefing paper and supporting documentation dated 7.5.2008, previously available on the EHTPA website.

[18] A copy of the letter between the HPC registrar and the Secretary of State for Health, previously available on the EHTPA website.

Practitioners of Western Herbal Medicine and Traditional Western Herbal Medicine who were members of the Unified Register of Herbal Practitioners (URHP) were not only discouraged from debating the issue on their members' forum; it was shut down under similar circumstances to the one hosted on the NIMH website; and all the relevant documentation was also removed from the members area of the website. In addition to this inhibition of debate, and the removal of the relevant documentation that might have helped individuals formulate their own opinion, the membership was also threatened, that if a member were to sign a petition against Statutory Regulation, the individual would be evicted from the Register.[19]

It should be remembered that it is only with some reluctance that the majority of practitioners had even accepted the idea of Statutory Self Regulation (SSR) in the first place.

This option was not even included in the WG on EPR Report. Statutory Regulation (SR) had been substituted in its place, although it had never been accepted by the majority of Herbalists. This inevitably launched the final Public Consultation Document on a somewhat uneven keel.

The proposal to statutory regulate Herbal Medicine, constitutes a de facto declaration that it is potentially so dangerous, that it could only be practised by state Registered professionals. This is the argument that has been put forward by the EHTPA to justify Statutory Regulation.[20]

The fact that the present empirical knowledge of Herbal Medicine has arisen from the traditional and cultural safe use over many thousands of years seems to disprove their point. The knowledge of traditional Herbal Medicine has been bestowed on mankind in every culture, in every land and on every continent of the world. It is a universal heritage that has been honed and adapted to meet the needs of mankind, wherever and in whatever

---

[19] E-mail to URHP members dated Tue, 14 Apr 2009 10:21

[20] Briefing Paper from the Chair of the European Herbal and Traditional Medicine Practitioners Association on the Statutory Regulation of Practitioners of Acupuncture, Herbal Medicine, Traditional Chinese Medicine and Other Traditional Medicine Systems practised in the UK, Document 3 (previously available on the EHTPA website)

circumstances he has found himself. It is owned by no one, but is the property of all.

The individual who was the guardian of this knowledge was also the shaman or priest of the community, who had a profound knowledge of the interconnection of the spiritual and physical realms. He, or indeed she, was acutely aware of the multi-dimensional facets of both their patients and the herbs, along with the procedures that they employed to treat the ills of both body and spirit. This knowledge is known to stretch back at least 5000 years in the annals of recorded history. It is the very length of the historical use that confirms Traditional Herbal Medicine as a matter of cultural significance within every society.

Herb residues, thought only to originate in South America, were even found amongst the burial goods of the ancient Egyptian mummies. Although this apparent anomaly might appear to raise more questions than it answers, it would appear to indicate a trans-global culture in Herbal Medicine that goes back through all the millennia of recorded history!

In comparatively recent times a great philosopher said:-

"The cure of the part should not be attempted without treatment of the whole.
No attempt should be made to cure the body without the soul, and if the head and the body are to be healthy, you must begin by curing the mind. For this is the greatest error of our day in the treatment of the human body, that the physicians separate the soul from the body." [21]

Unfortunately, since the time of the Cartesian divide, this separation between mind and body is precisely what has happened in the practice of modern Western Allopathic Medicine. Under the authority of a Papal Bull, the study of reductionist science became limited to only the physical aspects of man and the world in which he found himself.

---

[21] Plato 429 – 347 BC

To transgress this division became an act of heresy, which was seen not only to endanger the immortal soul, but also the mortal body, if the transgressor happened to get burned at the stake in recognition of his impertinence!

This dissociation between body and spirit has become a major source of disease, for which Traditional Herbal Medicine and its associated practices still remain the most potent cure. This is recognized by the WHO by its inclusion of the spiritual aspects of healing within its definition of traditional medicine and its recommendation that this should remain a source of primary healthcare.[22]

Comparatively recently, one of the foremost of the scientists of our time also confirmed his belief in the importance of the intangible aspects of creation, and their impact on mundane reality.

"Not everything that counts can be counted and not everything that can be counted counts." [23]

It must be taken into account however, that any paradigm exclusively dependent on reductionist science, is unable to consider or evaluate the relevance of the intangible. Similarly some religious belief systems may discount the existence of the human soul and the "life force" of the herb after it has been picked. On this basis, the World Health Organisation's definition of traditional medicine can potentially confront the belief systems of religion and science alike. In spite of these "confrontations" the philosophy of traditional Herbal Medicine recognizes these properties, and integrates them within its holistic practice.

The importance of the herb is also stated in both the Bible[24] and the Koran[25.] Although over the centuries both these religious tracts appear to have been subjected to vastly differing interpretations, the Bible text remains unchanged since the Nicene conference (325 AD), while other religious tracts have remained uncorrupted by political pressure.

---

[22] WHO Traditional Medicine Strategy 2002-2005 (page 13)

[23] Sign hanging in Einstein's office door at Princeton University

[24] further information available from
http://www.americancatholic.org/Newsletters/SFS/an0304.asp

[25] further information available from http://www.scribd.com/doc/17621/Remedies-From-the-Holy-QurAn

Because of this, it is held by some that any attempt to interfere with the accessibility of traditional Herbal Medicine would constitute an interference with their religious tradition and practice, and therefore a breach of their Civil Rights.

The traditional Herbal therapist developed many techniques to return stability and health to the patient. A naturopathic approach was seen as central to the treatment, as it was acknowledged that no regime, no matter how excellent in itself, would succeed if the patient continued to live in the way responsible for his illness. The traditional Herbalists developed a range of strategies that also included the use of acupuncture, acupressure, moxibustion and cupping (in the case of TCM) as well as Hopi ear candles, to name a few.

This range of activities, that have come to constitute the practice of traditional Herbal Medicine, must be borne in mind in considering the advice from the WG on EPR:-

"The scope of practice of the profession, or occupation, must have been agreed and defined.
If not, it will not be possible to pursue Statutory Regulation further, until such time as agreement about the function and scope of practice exists." [26]

Although stating the obvious, this is an extremely important admission, as without first defining the practice to be regulated, it would be impossible to regulate it.

The models for regulation were drawn up on a basis that had no regard to the diversities of practice within Traditional Western Herbal Medicine;[27] and that failure potentially threatens its future existence. As only one model of training has been recognized within the Steering Group Report, it has effectively produced a "one size fits all" approach that would be impossible to apply without fundamentally altering the very nature of the tradition.

---

[26] Interim Report from the Working Group on Extending Professional Regulation, Annexe E. 6.6.2008
[27] Report from the Working Group on Extending Professional Regulation 2009

This would be the inevitable result from the misapplication of inappropriate criteria, for the sole purpose of fitting the requirements to a fundamentally incompatible paradigm. Such an exercise, by its very nature would leave Traditional Herbal Medicine denatured and emasculated.

With its reduction to the status of an academic subject, future generations would become robbed of their heritage. As Traditional Herbal Medicine is an integral part of the National Heritage and Culture, any move to effectively crush its recognition and practise, would be in direct conflict with aspects of EU article 151 which states:-

"The community shall contribute to the flowering of the cultures of the Member states, while respecting their national and regional diversity and at the same time bringing the common heritage to the fore."
"The Community shall take cultural aspects into account in its action under other provisions of this Treaty, in particular in had order to respect and to promote the diversity of its cultures." [28]

We have now taken into account the historical development of traditional Herbal Medicine and its place in the various cultures of the world, and juxtaposed it with a number of diverse and contradictory reports.

It has become apparent that some of the documentation that has been put forward as supporting changes to the future regulation of Herbal Medicine, Acupuncture and Traditional Chinese Medicine, does not support the argument for any such change.

In the next chapter, the thorny question of defining Herbal Medicine in relation to this historical context and the catalogue of contradictory documentation, will be addressed.

***

---

[28] Communication from the Commission to the European Parliament, the Council, the European economic and Social Committee and the Committee of the Regions on a European agenda for culture in a globalizing world. Dated 14th May 2007

3

Defining Herbal Medicine

As stated previously: *"The scope of practice of the profession, or occupation, must have been agreed and defined. If not, it will not be possible to pursue Statutory Regulation further, until such time as agreement about the function and scope of practice exists."*[29]

This inevitably gives rise to the need to define Herbal Medicine and recognize the individuality of its varying traditions. During the process of compiling the Steering Group Report, a subtle but extremely serious "omission" occurred.

In the Report to Ministers from the Department of Health Steering Group on the Statutory Regulation of Practitioners of Acupuncture Herbal Medicine, Traditional Chinese Medicine and other Traditional Medicine Systems Practised in the UK, which was published in May 2008, there appeared to be a certain amount of confusion about the exact meaning of the term "Herbal Medicine."

The definition ultimately used was quite different from the description given in the EHTPA constitution. The significance of this is that the EHTPA Chairman sat as a "stakeholder chair" on the Steering Group Committee which drew up the report, and was therefore in a position to either correct or support the omission.

According to the Constitution of the European Herbal Traditional Practitioners Association (EHTPA), Herbal Medicine is described in the following way.

---

[29] Interim Report from the Working Group on Extending Professional Regulation, Annexe E. 6.6.2008

"Herbal Medicine"
The arts and sciences of any and all traditional or complementary systems of medicine (including but not limited to Traditional Chinese Medicine, Western Herbal Medicine, Ayurvedic Medicine and Traditional Tibetan medicine) and in which systems of medicine a main means of treatment is the provision of herbal medicines.
It is acknowledged that the definition of what constitutes herbal medicine may vary between Traditions and will reflect the legal position as laid down by the UK and EU medicines law and CITES.[30]

The clear implication here is that the variation in traditions would be recognized and taken into account within the proposals for regulation. As will be explained, this did not happen. In fact quite the opposite occurred, with the elimination of the recognition of the traditional Western paradigm, except, perhaps by default, by the phrase "including but not limited to".

Within the report itself **"Traditional Medicine"** was described as follows.

"WHO defines traditional medicine as follows: "Traditional medicine is a comprehensive term used to refer both to TM systems such as Traditional Chinese medicine, Indian Ayurveda and Arabic Unani medicine, and to various forms of indigenous medicine. TM therapies include medication therapies — if they involve use of herbal medicines, animal parts and/or minerals — and non-medication therapies — if they are carried out primarily without the use of medication, as in the case of acupuncture, manual therapies and spiritual therapies"[31]

Between these two statements we see a clear separation between Traditional Herbal Medicine and another non-traditional format which is subsequently referred to as Herbal Medicine within the report.

---

[30] (CITES: The Convention on International Trade in Endangered Species)
[31] Source WHO Traditional Med. Strategy 2002-2005 available at:
http://whqlibdoc.who.int/hq/2002/WHO_EDM_TRM_2002.1.pdf

It has already been explained that the modernist approach to Herbal Medicine differs fundamentally from that of practitioners of Traditional Herbal Medicine, to such a degree that they constitute two completely different schools of thought.

The traditional Herbalist evaluates the patient and his treatment on a holistic basis.
The traditional Herbalist works with the herb in its natural state, utilising his empirical knowledge of the effects of complex interactions of the constituent parts of the herb. The herb might be used "totum" either fresh or dried, or it might be used as a tea, decoction or as a tincture.

These are low intensity forms of delivery which are for the most part extremely safe. Herbal medicines used in traditional way also avoids challenging interactions with allopathic drugs. Traditional Herbal Medicine also works with the spirit, or subtle energy of the plant, and recognizes the interaction of the life force of the plant with that of the patient as an integral part of the treatment.

Therapies such as "Bach Flower Remedies" rely entirely on this aspect for their beneficial effect. Working in this way incorporates both the metaphysical and biochemical properties of herb.
This approach may give rise to different treatments for different patients, even though they may ostensibly present the same symptoms. This is the complete antithesis of the approach offered by allopathic medicine.

In the modernist (non-tradition) approach, the current teaching supports the use of concentrated extracts of the active biochemical component of the herb. The standardised extract is seen as delivering a standard reliable concentration of chemistry. This of course presents the digestive system of the patient with a concentration of biochemistry that does not occur in nature. Although this can be highly effective, it also runs the risk of raised levels of toxicity, which would have been negligible in the natural state.
Having been concentrated into what is in effect a pharmaceutical product, the potency of these preparations can on occasion give rise to troublesome interactions with similarly potent allopathic medications.

The modernist Herbalist, by virtue of working with a denatured pharmaceuticalized product, is no longer able to incorporate balanced and harmonious aspects of the life force from the original plant, and indeed consideration of this aspect becomes omitted altogether.

"For, as we maintain, it is only the addition or subtraction of the same substance from the same substance in the same order and in the same manner and in due proportion which will allow the latter to remain safe and sound in its sameness would itself.
But whatsoever oversteps any of these conditions in its going out it is coming in will produce alterations of every variety and countless diseases and corruptions."[32]

Translated into a more modern metaphor, the traditional Herbalist recognizes that the medicinal herb contains its own biochemical ecosystem, which becomes destructively unbalanced by the modernist use of the standardised extract. Plato demonstrates that this concept was already well understood over 2000 years ago.

In the non-traditional model the patient becomes regarded as merely being a collection of complex interactive biochemical processes. This approach mirrors that of allopathic medicine, and may perhaps be the result of the instruction of modernist Herbalists having been taken out of the hands of working herbalists, and put into those of university academics.

From this it follows that the philosophy behind the teaching of modernist Herbal Medicine and that of Traditional Herbal Medicine are separated at the extremes of a polarised spectrum. It is because of these essential differences that it would be totally inappropriate for them both to be incorporated under a single title.

These same differences of philosophy and approach also indicate that it might be possible for the modernist approach to reach some degree of accommodation within a regime, dominated by the philosophy and approach of allopathic medicine. The same could not be said of Traditional Herbal Medicine.

---

[32] Extract from Timaeus, by Plato.

Any attempt to force Traditional Herbal Medicine to comply with a set of criteria totally alien to its nature, would inevitably bring about the corruption of the tradition. This would obviously be to the detriment of Traditional Herbal Medicine as a discipline, to the detriment of the practitioner and to the detriment of the patient, who would have lost access to this vital modality of treatment.

It is this non-traditional format that claimed the title of "Herbal Medicine" for the purpose of pursuing Statutory Regulation.

The importance of this lies in the fact that regulation was being sought through the control of "protected title".

From this it would follow that <u>Traditional Herbal Medicine</u> would no longer come under the "protected title" of "Herbal Medicine". The Traditional Herbalists would become no longer legally allowed to call themselves Herbalists, and would have to adopt a new un-protected title.

As previously stated, this has already happened with non statutory regulated Osteopaths.

A change of title would inevitably give rise to a high degree of confusion amongst the public. Confusions of this kind could only result in the effective loss of access to Traditional Herbal Medicine. This in turn would be to the detriment of the interests of the public and practitioner alike.

Here we are again reminded that one of the proposed benefits of Statutory Regulation, as advocated by the HPC, is the protection of the traditions. In the above scenario, the exact opposite would be the effect.

The effective redefinition of Herbal Medicine was proposed in the following manner. The Steering Group Report suggested that the distribution of "title" should be as follows in the diagram below, clearly indicating the inclusion of a diversity of approaches and traditions.

This was almost in line with the definitions laid down by the World Health Organisation, but not quite.....

GENERIC	TRADITION	TITLE
Herbal/ Traditional Medicine Practitioner	Ayurveda	Ayurvedic Practitioner
	Traditional Chinese Medicine	Traditional Chinese Medicine Practitioner
		Chinese Herbal Medicine Practitioner
	Traditional Tibetan Medicine	Traditional Tibetan Medicine Practitioner
	Unani Tibb	Unani Tibb Practitioner
	Western Herbal Medicine	Herbalist
		Western Herbal Medicine Practitioner
		Medical Herbalist

On the left of the table, the concept of Traditional Herbal Medicine would appear to be all-inclusive.

Closer examination of the table, however, demonstrates that the traditional aspects of Chinese and Tibetan Medicine are recognised, but no mention is made to the existence of a Western Tradition, (The title of 'Traditional Western Herbal Medicine Practitioner), the practitioners of which would therefore become excluded from the right to use the protected title 'Herbalist' in any of its generic forms.

There are major differences, as described above, between Traditional Western Herbal Medicine, which uses the herb in its natural state, and the modernist non-traditional Herbal Medicine with a preference for a laboratory produced semi pharmaceutical product, which does not occur in nature.

As this divergence between two very differing traditions was not recognized, it was not catered for in the promise:

"It is acknowledged that the definition of what constitutes herbal medicine may vary between Traditions and will reflect the legal position as laid down by the UK and EU medicines law and CITES".[33]

The modernists only separated from the traditionalists, with their millennia of experience, during the middle part of the 20th-century. In spite of this, the move to give them control of the "protected title", and therefore the exclusive right to use it, would legally deny it to its historic guardians and rightful heirs, the Traditional (Western) Herbalist.

The cuckoo hatchling would therefore have succeeded in ejecting the legitimate chicks from the nest and claiming it as its own.

As a result of this, the traditional aspects of Herbal Medicine would henceforth only be recognized in the eastern traditions.

The acceptance of the Eastern traditions did however give official recognition to the subtle energy aspects that are also an inherent part of Western traditional practice.

NB[1]. The EHTPA Chairman sat as a stakeholder member on the Steering Group Committee, and admitted having a major influence over its content.[34]

The EHTPA Chairman is a member of NIHM which advocates the modernist approach to Herbal Medicine and is also a member of the Register of Chinese Herbal Medicine. It is therefore possible that the defining aspects of <u>Traditional</u> Western Herbal Medicine may not have been adequately represented on the Committee that drew up the Steering Group Report.

Subtle energy and the spiritual aspects of the herb are not recognized in modern reductionist science. Without this recognition it could not be taught

---

[33] Quote from the EHTPA constitution.

[34] Briefing paper to the Minister of State for Health Services and associated documentation dated 7.5.2008, previously available on the EHTPA website

as part of a science degree course, as specified as a requirement for HPC regulation.

NB[2]. In the event of Statutory Regulation being introduced, under grandparenting arrangements, <u>existing</u> experienced practitioners could theoretically be adopted, irrespective of their tradition or training. This however would not apply after the closing of a brief window of opportunity.

Under this regime, the current generation of traditional herbal practitioners would also become the last to be able to practise under their traditional title. Even those who might have made the transition to HPC regulation, to continue under that regime would have to "upgrade" their training to fit a model alien to their craft.

The treatments given by a Traditional Western Herbalist will inevitably vary from those given by a Traditional Tibetan practitioner, a Traditional Ayurvedic practitioner or a Traditional Chinese practitioner.

In spite of these variations of practice however, in many ways the basic philosophies of these traditions would show a far greater degree of compatibility than would be the case with the philosophy of the modernist approach.

Although the traditional aspects could be studied as a postgraduate addition to the modernist training, their practice would fall outside the defined model of regulated practice.

Because of this, a regulated practitioner utilising the traditional protocols, might find himself in a vulnerable position, accused of unprofessional, or even superstitious practice. Here we are reminded of the narrow confines of reductionist science, as laid down by the Cartesian divide described earlier.

This disparity will be further discussed in the next chapter.

***

4

Disparity in Evidence of Efficacy

One of the specific criteria that need to be fulfilled to qualify for HPC regulation is,

"Practice based on evidence of efficacy."[35]

For Traditional Herbal Medicine this is something of a thorny issue. The problem does not lie with the issue of efficacy, but with the problem of precisely what does, or does not constitute "evidence". We are told that in situations such as this, the term "evidence" denotes that which can be discerned and proved by (reductionist) science.

The majority of Herbal Medicine Traditions have a knowledge base gained from some 5,000 years of empirical experience. However, in the eyes of reductionist science, this is not deemed acceptable, as it only demonstrates that something does work and not how. It would, however, be interesting for a pharmaceutical company to answer the question about exactly how many of its products had been subjected to such extensive field trials!

On page 10 of The Steering Group Report it was stated that one of the HPC criteria for SR was that the area of activity should be based on a "Practice based on evidence of efficacy."

This continues to present a problem to the champions of Statutory Regulation.

---

[35] information available on the HPC website at http://www.hpc-uk.org/aboutregistration/newprofessions/criteria/

In the Steering Group Report there was an interesting discussion as to what did or did not constitute "evidence".

Within this presentation, that which can only be described as empirical knowledge apparently became accepted as "evidence".

Paradoxically, it was subsequently suggested that TCM should be promoted for Statutory Regulation under <u>level 3.</u> The description given to <u>level 3</u> on the EHTPA website was <u>"having no evidence base for clinical effectiveness."</u> [36]

One of the problems has always been that part of the paradigm in which Herbal Medicine functions, lies completely outside the areas covered by reductionist science. This makes it a totally inappropriate tool to measure its efficacy.

The difference in the criteria for establishing efficacy is one of the major reasons why the Traditional Herbal Medicine of any culture should not come under the same jurisdiction as Western allopathic medicine.

While, at the same time as admitting this discrepancy in what constitutes evidence of efficacy[37], the RCHM (Register of Chinese Herbal Medicine) is proposing that Statutory Regulation should go ahead without the evidence base having been developed.

"When it comes to older treatments, there is often a gap between empirical evidence, clinical practice, and patient experience. Moreover, there are conspicuous double standards in attitudes to older treatments. For example, about half of all so-called conventional healthcare interventions continue to be used even though research on their efficacy is non-existent or equivocal.
By contrast, traditional complementary and alternative therapies that have been widely used for many years and continue to be popular with patients are regularly dismissed out of hand on the grounds that there is little 'scientific' evidence to confirm whether they work". [38]

---

[36] Information formerly posted on the EHTPA website

[37] See RCHM official response to public consultation questionnaire.

[38] Extract from RCHM response to question 12 the public consultation questionnaire

There are also obvious problems associated with focusing entirely on published trial literature as the supposed basis for evidence-based practice.

The efficacy studies that form the backbone of EBM[39] represent only a small part of the total research literature, and may be of limited value in assessing safety.

And, of course, most efficacy research is sponsored by the pharmaceutical industry and is drug orientated. Potentially valuable traditional medicines, non-drug interventions, or other aspects of health care receive much less attention."

Even the House of Lords Select Committee on Science and Technology stated that Acupuncture and Herbal Medicine only had an "incomplete evidence base".[40]

This is rather like saying, "I did quite well during the first 10 minutes of my driving test, but unfortunately I didn't complete it. It does not matter that I did not complete the test, I still want my driving license anyway!"

If inappropriate terms of reference are used to evaluate traditional Herbal Medicine, it can only lead to such a distortion of the traditional approach that it would effectively cease to exist.

As has been confirmed above, even those organisations that officially advocate their own Statutory Regulation, confirmed that they do not comply with the required terms of reference.

This returns us yet again to the concept of destruction of the tradition by regulation, and not its protection, as is claimed by the HPC. This would seem to indicate that the application for HPC regulation is one driven by desperation rather than enthusiasm.

***

---

[39] Evidence Based Medicine

[40] As quoted in the EHTPA briefing paper and associated documentation dated 7.5.2008 to Mr Ben Bradshaw Minister of State for Health Services, and posted on the EHTPA website.

5

Models of Regulation

The Working Group on Extending Professional Regulation produced an excellent and concise report which discussed this subject at length in Appendix D.

It should be borne in mind that the report was drawn up to cover a much wider range of activities than those involved in the practice of Herbal Medicine and was primarily concerned with activities carried out within the NHS.

"For the NHS in England, professional regulation will have an important enabling and assuring role to play in delivering the quality improvement and health improvement agenda set out in the Next Stage Review. Likewise, implementation of quality service delivery strategies in each of the Devolved Administrations rely on a workforce that is well prepared and fit for purpose."[41]

The Working Group on Extending Professional Regulation report can be downloaded as a PDF file from:-
http://www.dh.gov.uk/en/Publicationsandstatistics/Publications/Publicat
ionsPolicyAndGuidance/DH_102824

One thing that becomes immediately obvious is that the report encompasses a wide range of options, and discusses their relative strengths and weaknesses. Unfortunately some Professional Association members of the EHTPA focused exclusively on the most draconian option, Statutory Regulation, and did so to the exclusion of all others.

---

[41] Extract from the introduction to WG on EPR report it

This obsession appears to have left them unable even to publicly admit the very existence of the concept of choice in this matter, although the Government has repeatedly stated that it has been considering several models of regulation in search of the most appropriate one.[42] Unlike the Steering Group Report, *(see box below)*, the submission from the WG on EPR is a work of both detail and clarity.

The SR obsessives have openly taken to complaining that they have been unable to comprehend a simplified document that makes up the Public Consultation Document, which can be downloaded as a PDF file from:-

http://www.dh.gov.uk/en/Consultations/Liveconsultations/DH0

This particular interest group has even posted a pre- formatted postcard which they have urged their followers to copy, which openly states that:-

a. The ability to fill out public consultation questionnaire is beyond their intellectual means and

b. That despite their inability to master the complexities, they have still decided that Statutory Regulation is the only acceptable option.

c. The concept of "decision-making and choice" involves an act of "informed consent". To be informed, presupposes the ability to comprehend.

Here it should be acknowledged that the DOH has distanced itself from responsibility for the "Steering Group" report, by emphasizing that it was a report "to Government" from an independent body, and not a Government report.

(Sharon Corner, European & Specialist Legislation Team, Workforce Directorate, Dept. of Health 26.6.2008)

This basic requirement seems to have escaped consideration.

---

[42] E.g. Letter from Kate Roy, Customer Service Centre Dept. of Health 16.12.2008, the WG on EPR report and the Public Consultation Document

It is a further matter of concern that in some cases, this concept of "uninformed consent" seems to have to be been advocated by members of the higher echelons of those same professional bodies, at a level commensurable with EHTPA directorship.

Advice to the public, proposing a request based on "uninformed consent" has been posted on an EHTPA Professional Association website, in the form of a pre-formatted postcard requesting Statutory Regulation, which stated:-

As consumer, I want the Government to establish Statutory Regulation for Herbal Medicine, Acupuncture, TCM and other traditional medicine systems.

No other arrangement than Statutory Regulation will meet my needs.

I could not fill in the Consultation response online due to its complexity and difficulty of use.43

Caveat emptor
(Buyer Beware)

"Buyer Beware" is probably the most authentic warning that has ever applied to any practitioner, either in parallel to, or independently from any other regulatory paradigm under which they might operate. Those who have a reputation for excellence attract the business of potential patients. Those of a less magnificent reputation do not.

In ancient China it was the custom for the medical practitioner to be paid for maintaining the health of the patient, rather than for his ministrations during sickness. The doctor was therefore seen as a "health" practitioner rather than a "sickness" practitioner, which has unfortunately become the role of those working in allopathic medicine.

The allopathic model seeks to compensate for the dysfunction of the body. Traditional medicine seeks to correct the ailment by correcting its cause,

---

43 Extract from pre-formatted postcard downloaded, publically available from the URHP website

thereby promoting natural health rather than its synthetic parody that has a marked tendency to shorten life expectancy. Under this traditional paradigm of practice, the successful practitioner thrived, while the natural selection of the marketplace drove the unsuccessful out of business.

The **Caveat Emptor** model of regulation is therefore based on public awareness. As a significant proportion of any Medical Herbalists' patient list is achieved through the process of personal recommendation, his or her ability to remain in business is totally dependent on the skill to maintain a reputation for successful outcomes.

Within this model, the public is already protected by a whole raft of consumer protection legislation and criminal law.

Traditional Western Herbalists Practitioners, currently operating under the current provisions and/or under the historic protection that had been afforded them by Henry VIII, have done so without posing any significant risk to the public and without the imposition of either statutory, or any other form of legally enforced regulation. The concept, that the status of the Herbal practitioner is already regulated by public acclaim and his standing in the community, is even reflected in the WHO report on the future of traditional medicine.

Wherever failures may have occurred, this has been due to the lack of implementation of existing legislation, consumer protection, and trading standards, 12.1 of the Herbalist Act, laws relating to common assault etc. and not its lack of existence. Any argument that further legislation is called for cannot be substantiated. "If it ain't broke, why fix it?"

One of the major attractions to this traditional approach is that it allows the therapist to employ a full range of strategies at his or her own command, in line with the definition described by the World Health Organisation.

This model recognizes the Herbalist as a healer, guide and holistic therapist, and not just a merchandiser of laboratory produced botanical products.

Many therapists have gained their professional reputations through the practice of excellence in specific areas of interest. As a result of this, they have accumulated multiple but diverse collections of strategies.

This diversity, while being the product of their expertise, would also present problems to any regime of regulation based on "tick the box" categorisation. It is this very diversity that would be disastrously endangered by the imposition of a narrowly defined "discreet and homogenous" area of activity, as laid down as a basic requirement for Statutory Regulation by the HPC.

The concept of "cloned" therapists is the very antithesis of diversity and choice. The protection of diversity is <u>theoretically</u> championed by the European Union.

"The community shall contribute to the flowering of the cultures of the Member states, while respecting their national and regional diversity and at the same time bringing the common heritage to the fore."
"The Community shall take cultural aspects into account in its action under other provisions of this Treaty, in particular in had order to respect and to promote the diversity of its cultures." [44]

The philosophy of individuality would similarly sit somewhat uncomfortably in any regime based on the compliance with uniformity. Here it should be borne in mind that the WG on EPR report, excellent in itself, was written from the world view of the NHS.

"For the NHS in England, professional regulation will have an important enabling and assuring role to play in delivering the quality improvement and health improvement agenda set out in the Next Stage Review. Likewise, implementation of quality service delivery strategies in each of the Devolved Administrations rely on a workforce that is well prepared and fit for purpose." [45]

This world view, all too often, has a tendency to look back at itself through rose tinted glasses.

---

[44] Communication from the Commission to the European Parliament, the Council, the European economic and Social Committee and the Committee of the Regions on a European agenda for culture in a globalizing world. Dated 14th May 2007.
[45] WG on EPR Report (page 5)

Institutionally it is in denial of the gross failings that are often the product of Government regulation and the "tick the box" approach to which it gives rise.

Over the years, Government regulation has notoriously given rise to a top-heavy burden of bureaucracy, the funding of which has increasingly drawn cash away from the actual delivery of care.

"It is time for a serious evaluation of unaccountable self-serving administrative structures that sideline doctors and nurses and impede patient care."[46]

The move towards "professionalism" in nursing, with the requirement for university degree qualifications, has already attracted a degree of criticism. There have been well publicised fears that progressive professionalisation will redefine the role of nursing away from personal care, towards the technical administration of clinical procedures. With this change of emphasis in the role of the nurse, many of the traditional functions have already become delegated to lower ranking auxiliaries.

The maintenance of the hygiene of the hospital has often been given out on tender to the company offering the cheapest provision. This in turn has led to several much publicised crises with hospital wards having to be shut down for "deep cleaning", to deal with the MRSA crisis. In the Times, on the 17th of December 2009, it was reported on page 16 that NHS unions had complained that doctors and nurses at Alder Hey children's hospital in Liverpool had been asked to help clean the wards prior to inspection by the Care Quality Commission.

This highlights the problems that have already occurred through the limitations imposed by the requirement to define the parameters of activity of the purposes of regulation and the pursuit of professional status. Vulnerable patients have been left unfed, requiring members of the family to attend the hospital at mealtimes to care for their loved ones, who are too frail to feed themselves. All of this makes a mockery of the argument that

---

[46] Jonathon Waxman, Professor of Oncology at Imperial College London, the Times newspaper 17.12.2009 (page 34)

professionalisation through regulation gives rise to an improvement in standards, and promotes public safety.

It is the independent practitioner of Herbal Medicine that all too often is required to treat the victims of the state regulated "Health" Service. If for no other reason than this, it remains an absolute imperative that Herbal Medicine should continue to be allowed to thrive, independent of control by any organisation dominated by the philosophy and practice of Western allopathic medicine. As has been demonstrated above, regulation not only fails to produce the raising of standards, but may even hinder the maintenance of existing ones, by siphoning off essential funding for the purposes of administration.

In the eventuality of the "caveat emptor" model being maintained, the WG on EPR recommended appropriate information should be made available to members of the public, so that they may be able to evaluate the most appropriate course of therapy for them.

Access to open and accurate information would allow the public to give meaningful informed consent to any provision offered. In order for such meaningful informed consent to be given, logically this ought to include the open admission of the risks posed by allopathic medicine, so that risk comparison analysis can be made.

Much of this information is available and published annually in the MIMS manual. The known risks and contraindications of allopathic drugs published in this manual are often not taken into account by allopathic practitioners. This same information however it routinely used by Herbalists to identify the source of the health problems presented to them by their patients.

It is in the job of the Herbalist to report back to their patient's doctor that it is the allopathic prescription that is causing the current health problem, as responsibility for the prescription lies with the allopathic practitioner.

The statistical evidence that might be made available to members of the public, to help them to make informed decisions, should also relate to conventional medicine. This would offer a comparison of risk between the options available.

E.g.- *"Of around 2500 [commonly used NHS] treatments covered 13% are rated as beneficial, 23% likely to be beneficial, 8% as trade off between benefits and harms, 6% unlikely to be beneficial, 4% likely to be ineffective or harmful, and 46%, the largest proportion, as unknown effectiveness."*[47]

In the decade up to 2007, 80,000 people were reported to have died from adverse side effects of their medication, with a further £46,000,000 being spent by the NHS to treat the side effects of the survivors.[48]

"An extraordinary rise in the number of patients killed by drugs given out by the health service has led to calls for an investigation.

The figure has more than doubled since Labour came to power rising from 520 in 1998 to 1299 last year.

Official figures also show that the number of such deaths last year was up by more than a quarter of the figure of 1,030 recorded in 2007." [49]

Here the reader is reminded that the proposed level of regulation is required to be proportional to risk.

According to the Actuary Tables of risk used by Balens, the premier insurance company for complementary and alternative medicine, Herbalism poses a similar level of risk to Astrology, Crystal Therapy and Creative Writing. It would therefore be totally inappropriate for Herbal Medicine to come under anything like the same level of regulation as that of allopathic medicine, or even the same regulator! The current death rates from allopathic drugs further indicate how biased and unreliable the MHRA recommendations for the approval of drugs actually are. This subject will be covered in more depth in a later chapter.

---

[47] BMJ Evidence Centre http://clinicalevidence.bmj.com/ceweb/about/knowledge.jsp

[48] Article by Jenny Hope, medical correspondent (Daily Mail)

[49] From an article written in 2009 entitled "Why is NHS killing so many with drugs?" By Daniel Martin Health Reporter (Daily Mail)

"**Caveat Emptor**" would be the most appropriate option for the independent Herbalist, as it does not involve the expense of Government regulation, and this would not then have to be passed on to the patient. "Caveat emptor" is the model under which Herbal Medicine has traditionally been practised for over 5000 years.

Voluntary Self-Regulation

Voluntary Self-Regulation was the original preferred option of the Professional Associations making up the membership of the European Herbal Traditional Practitioners Association. The argument, from the start, was a fear that Statutory Regulation might eventually be imposed by the Government, unless a viable alternative regime of regulation could be arrived at. This, it was hoped, would ward off the unacceptable threat to Herbal Medicine in its diverse traditions.

It has since emerged that this "threat" cannot be substantiated, as the HPC has clearly stated that Statutory Regulation is something for which the "aspirant" would have to apply, and the "threat" that it might be involuntarily imposed, should therefore be discounted. It would therefore seem that the EHTPA has not only set about providing the solution to a non-existent problem, but has in fact relentlessly kept the issue alive by actively pursuing Statutory Regulation itself. This has been a direct contradiction to the terms under which it initially recruited its membership. The EHTPA has made inferences about the alleged democratic support for this reversal of policy[50,] which are difficult to substantiate numerically.

One of the largest member organisations, or Professional Associations (PAs), of NIMH members, only 28% voted for regulation at the last EGM. 68% of members did not vote. Similar figures have been the case ever since regulation became a voting issue. On discussing this with members who did not vote, many of them said it was because they felt they had not been given sufficient information to make an informed decision, and the information they did receive was confusing.

---

[50] EHTPA Briefing paper and associated documentation dated 7.5.2008 to Mr Ben Bradshaw Minister of State for Health Services, previously available on the EHTPA website.

The membership of another EHTPA PA, the Unified Register of Herbal Practitioners (URHP), was threatened by e-mail (*Sent: Tue, 14 Apr 2009 10:21*) with expulsion from the Register if they signed a petition against Statutory Regulation being applied to Herbal Medicine.

Debate amongst the membership of these two Registers, about this change of policy became restricted by the decision to shut down the member's discussion forums on both their websites.

In these circumstances, it is difficult to maintain the illusion of democratic approval for this measure.

The membership of another Register, the International Register of Consultant Herbalists and Homoeopaths (IRCH) was never consulted on this change of policy. The IRCH has since resigned from the EHTPA on the grounds that current EHTPA policy is not in the best interests of either the IRCH itself or future interests of Traditional Herbal Medicine in general.

In the light of the above information, it is arguable that, in the absence of Statutory Self- Regulation as an option, **Voluntary Self Regulation** should remain the official preference of the **EHTPA**, in response to the public consultation document. Unfortunately, quite the contrary impression was given in the correspondence between the EHTPA Chairman and the then Minister of Health, Mr Ben Bradshaw, in the official exchanges of correspondence on this subject.

In the documentation that was sent to Mr Bradshaw by the Chairman of the EHTPA, a number of facts and figures were presented that gave the illusion of wholesale support for the introduction of Statutory Regulation of Herbal Medicine.

Great play was made of the percentage of approval given by a previous consultation on this subject (98.5% in favour), but on further examination of the correspondence it was revealed that the total number of votes cast on this subject only amounted to **698**.

Making full use of the wonders of modern technology (a pocket calculator), even the most mathematically inept may be able to deduce that the number of votes cast in favour of this proposition only amounted to **687.53**[51]

Although there is noticeably little information about the status of the individual who was only accredited **0.53** of a vote, this does give rise to some interesting questions.

On which hypothesis did this partial validity of vote stand?

a.   Was the individual a multiple amputee, and if so, how did this detract from the validity of his/her vote? If this had been the case, it would have been an infringement of the individual's civil rights.

b.   Was the individual only 0 .53% human? This would have indicated that the individual was some sort of trans-species chimera.

c.   Are the statistics as incompetent as they are misleading?

In any event this hardly amounted to a national mandate to fundamentally alter the legal status of the provision of Herbal Medicine, whether of a traditional paradigm, or not. There remains a number of questions about exactly how many people were actually involved in the consultation, what was the nature of their interest in the subject and what was the accuracy, balance and scope of the information that they were given upon which to base their opinions. In the light of the latest public consultation, all these questions are particularly relevant!

Voluntary Self-Regulation allows the professional body to lay down the appropriate level of training that is proportionate to the area of activity. As VSR is carried out under the banner of a professional Register, it presupposes the requirement of a constitution and code of ethics. As membership of the Register is seen as the assurance of excellence, it is in the interest of the Register to control and maintain the standards of its membership.

---

[51] EHTPA Briefing paper and associated documentation dated 7.5.2008 to Mr Ben Bradshaw Minister of State for Health Services, previously available on the EHTPA website.

Voluntarily self regulated Registers have the power to discipline their members through the implementation of their constitutional complaints procedure. This presents any miscreants with the threat of being deregulated from the Register, together with a debarment from being able to use any style or title controlled by the Register. This disciplinary outcome is already similar to that offered by Statutory Regulation.

Because of this, Voluntary Self-Regulation provides an equitable surety of protection to the public, in this respect.

The WG on EPR report suggested that a private Register, being effectively owned by the membership ran the risk of being lax about maintaining standards.

As has been pointed out above, any acts that fail in maintaining standards would effectively undermine the good name of the Register, and be counter to its own interests. As an example of this, the MHRA (which is supposed to regulate products of the pharmaceutical companies) has been found to be so lax in its regulatory duties, that its suspension from the Department of Health has already been recommended.[52]

This will be discussed in more depth in a later chapter.

In the light of the examples of Nurse Beverley Allit (RCN) and Dr Harold Shipman (BMA), there is no evidence to support any claim that Statutory Regulation would be any more effective than Voluntary Self-Regulation in protecting the public.

In point of fact, no regulatory regime, no matter how authoritarian, is capable of restraining the conduct of any of its members, but is only able to apply disciplinary measures after the event.

The Working Group Report expressed concern that, under VSR, a debarred registrant might continue to practise, and that competing Registers might be set up with differing standards and rules. In practice however, applicants to

---

[52] House of Commons Health Committee Report from 2005, entitled 'The Influence of the Pharmaceutical Industry

Registers are required to sign a declaration about any complaints that might have been made about them, and their outcomes.

If misinformation is provided, and subsequently exposed, the applicant becomes expelled from the Register.

As already stated, it is in the self interest of each and every Register and its membership to maintain its own good name, so this concern about VSR not being the appropriate level of regulation cannot be maintained at more than a notional level.

Even in the case of Statutory Regulation, a disbarred practitioner would still be able to practice under an alternative title, as HPC regulation is by "protected title", not function.

This consideration alone might be seen to make the supposed authority the Independent Safeguarding Authority (and equivalent regimes) less relevant than anticipated. In this area again, VSR offers as much public protection as SR but without excessive burden of expense involved in the latter.

It was noted that as the subsequent WG on EPR reports were based on the initial recommendations in the Steering Group Report, some of its inconsistent and paradoxical nature became reflected in them.

On the one hand it was stated in the Interim Report from the WG on EPR that:-

"Assuming all other criteria have been met, the suitability of non-statutory forms of regulation should have been considered and there should be a compelling argument for transferring any existing system of non-Statutory Regulation to a statutory system." [53]

But in the final report from the WG on EPR, it was suggested that VSR might be seen as a staging post for Statutory Regulation.

---

[53] The Interim Report from the WG on EPR, page 26

Voluntary Self Regulation

This model is already widely adopted by many unregulated professional and occupational groups within health care as <u>a</u> <u>preparatory stage prior to Statutory Regulation.</u>

The Working Group considered that by providing more robust and consistent approaches to voluntary registration with a stronger degree of assurance and accreditation, the approach of a voluntary registration regime could play a valuable part in the overall system of regulation.

The Working Group recommends that the Department of Health in England and the Devolved Administrations work with the CHRE,[54] and other key stakeholders to consider the costs, benefits, and feasibility of developing a formal voluntary accreditation regime to supplement voluntary Registers within the menu of regulatory choices.[55]

If VSR was seen to be adequate and appropriate to requirements, by definition SR would be inappropriate, as the degree of regulation is determined by the level of risk posed to the public, and not by the professional aspiration of the applicant! At the time of writing, this inherent contradiction remains unresolved.

Given the multiplicity of smaller traditions, each with their own unique identity, VSR offers the benefits of inexpensive regulation coupled with the inherent adaptability that is required to match the level and type(s) of training that are relevant to the tradition itself.

Voluntary Self-Regulation is the appropriate option for groups of Herbalists wishing to maintain the independent identity of their particular traditional paradigm of Herbal Medicine, while at the same time offering a level of surety of excellence to the public, supported by the membership of a professional Register.

---

[54] Council for Healthcare Regulatory Excellence

[55] The WG on EPR Report

The case for voluntary self-regulation being appropriate for traditional herbal medicine is largely substantiated by the WG on EPR report. This is the level of regulation promoted as being the appropriate one for Naturopathy and Nutritional Therapy.[56]

As these two therapeutic approaches form the backbone of traditional herbal medicine, it is questionable that a more stringent approach would be supportable under the criteria of regulation needing to be proportional to risk. The absence of a need to statutory regulate traditional herbal medicine, for the purposes of harmonisation with European legislation, is further indicated by the statement in the WG on EPR report, under the subheading "European Regulation".

"Even if the occupation or profession of the immigrant health care worker is not regulated in their home state but is in the host state, provided they can provide suitable evidence that they have been practising their profession in their home state they may have a right to be entered on the register of the host state, subject to making up any shortfalls in training or experience.
The Working Group recognised that their proposals would need to be consistent with EU requirements."[57]

Employer led regulation

This model of regulation received two and a half pages of discussion in the WG on EPR Report. As previously stated, the WG on EPR Report primarily relates to those employed in the NHS. By definition this format of regulation provides public protection through a code of conduct that applies to employees working in health care support. This format of regulation could not be relevant to the self employed professional, and could only come into force if a Medical Herbalist were to take up employment in the NHS, as a Medical Herbalist.

---

[56] Page 34 WG on EPR report
[57] Page 42 WG on EPR report

This would presuppose the NHS accepting Herbal Medicine as an "approved therapy", and categorising it as "care support".

A scheme was piloted in Scotland in three NHS Boards and one Independent Hospital. For the purposes of the pilot scheme, "Health Care Support Workers" involved those in direct contact with patients and members of the public in the name of NHS Scotland. This covered a range of employees with widely differing degrees of contact with patients.

The approval rating for the universal Statutory Regulation of this highly variable body of employees came in at 93% of a 90% response. The universality, in the degree and nature of regulation, obviously simplifies its administration, and would therefore provide financial savings. Although the figures quoted show a considerable degree of compliance with the administrative interests of the employer, they also give rise to some interesting questions in the enquiring mind of a student of human nature.

1) In a culture of voter apathy, how was such a high level of voter turn-out achieved, despite the natural attrition on numbers by sickness, injury, holiday leave and a statistically probable level of domestic or personal problems that would delegate issues such as this outside the parameters of voter routes?

2) How was that vote taken? Was it by the genuine secret ballot, or by public show of hands? The latter is notorious for its ability to be manipulated by peer pressure and the authority of the individual(s) conducting the ballot.

3) Was the option of regulation presented as the lesser of two or more "evils", one or other of which would be imposed upon the workforce in any case?

4) Was the acceptance of regulation tied into a pay benefit that was dependent upon it?

5) Was consideration given to the inescapable fact that any form of regulation of the individual for the benefit of the public, can only be

achieved by imposing an extra level of vulnerability on the regulated individual?

6) This would have to take into account the unfortunate fact that there are a number of individuals in the community from whom the regulated practitioner actually needs protecting; that is:-

   a. Those who take delight in exercising the ability to exert fear and control over others.

   b. Those who make false complaints in pursuit of compensation or in the hope of being bought off with an out-of-court settlement.

   c. Those that seek public notoriety, and see "victimhood" as a way of achieving it.

   d. Psychologically disturbed individuals, who by virtue of their condition, "project" the responsibility for their previous traumatic experience on to the regulated individual.

   e. Those with a pathological sense of grievance against members of the profession.

Although disciplinary and complaint procedures are an essential part of the regulatory package, and these provide the system through which inappropriate complaints can be resolved, they can in no way either un-do, or compensate the falsely accused of the trauma from the experience involved.

In agreeing to be regulated, the individual must, by necessity, accept the suspension of the sword Damocles over his head, with the level of regulation determining the stoutness of the thread.

Although this form of regulation would not apply to a self employed professional practitioner, the concerns stated above must equally apply to all models of regulation, except of course one based on "caveat emptor" (buyer beware).

It may perhaps be significant that the model of regulation piloted in Scotland does not have the support of the Trade Unions which represent health care support workers across the UK!

It should also be noted that the cohort which piloted the scheme amounted to only 1/6 of those eligible in Scotland.[58]

Although the figures quoted in the report are doubtlessly scrupulously accurate, in light of the above it would be unsafe to assume that they in any way demonstrate the acceptability of the provision across the full spectrum to which it might be applied.

Similarly, they should not be used to support the notion of acceptability for any other level of regulation for any other group.

For those with an academic interest in this subject, the information can be found on pages 36-38 of the WG on EPR Report. Although it is not envisaged that Herbal Medicine, Acupuncture or traditional Chinese Medicine would ever become subject to this form of regulation, consideration should be given to the inherent vulnerabilities (as listed above) that would be inevitably visited upon the practitioner under any form of state controlled regulation.

It is well worth asking the question whether or not the debate on the subject of Statutory Regulation has ever included these points for consideration!

Licensing

Within the WG on EPR Report, the discussion was interesting, but purely hypothetical and undecided about the exact structure it might take. This makes the proposition somewhat difficult to evaluate. The basic issue remains the comparative efficacy of one form of regulation in comparison to another, to achieve three core objectives.

---

[58] WG on EPR Report, Page 37, Paras. 4.34 & 4.35

1. To ensure appropriate standards based training/qualifications for the role;

2. To help secure adherence to a code of conduct; and,

3. To ensure that those, whose conduct does not meet the required standards, are barred from carrying out these roles in the future.

The Report was uncertain as to whether it should offer a single uniform standard of licensing, or a group of licences that reflect the different levels of risk presented by different occupational roles. This admission of uncertainty seems to present something of a paradox, in that it juxtaposes two conflicting statements.

1) There is already a statement that the degree of regulation should be relevant to risk.

2) This model was potentially considering applying the same level of regulation, in relation to occupations offering different levels of risk.[59]

The powers of the licensing bodies have yet to be defined. Without that definition it remains impossible to evaluate how viable or appropriate this form of regulation might be.

4.41 A licensing body or bodies (yet to be defined), could hold a list of names of licensed workers who had met the necessary requirements for their role and signed up to the relevant code of conduct.

Licences could, for example, be removed following complaint and investigation at a tribunal and, if licensees wished to be reinstated, their appeals could be heard in the appropriate Court in England and the corresponding competent Court within the Devolved Administration jurisdictions as appropriate.

---

[59] WG on EPR Report, Page 39, Para. 4.40

On a more positive note this section returned to the notion that the degree of regulation should be proportional to risk.

4.42 Licensing could be either mandatory, required by statute, or voluntary and dependent upon employers requiring licensure as a condition of employment. The precise form of licensing vehicle would be dependent on the risk posed by the activity and the most proportionate manner required to protect the public from risk.

The Security Industry Authority is one example of this regime operating in another sector.[60]

This potential HPC model was described as being potentially either:-

"mandatory, required by statute, or voluntary and dependent upon employers requiring licensure as a condition of employment" [61]

It was later described as being:-

"a quasi- voluntary regime dependent on market forces making licensed workers a key hallmark of quality, but compulsion could be introduced through statutory licensing regimes."[62]

Given the undecided and variable nature of this proposition, it would be impossible to advocate its adoption without a great deal of further clarification. Although it was described as having "considerable attractions" through it's essentially chameleon like characteristics, it is these very characteristics that make it impossible to evaluate in any meaningful way.

If and when a more clearly defined proposal were to be made available for consideration, it might well be worth investigating further.
It should be mentioned here that this was one of a raft of proposals from the WG on EPR to the Secretary of State for consideration.
Without a clearly defined model having been presented, he would not have been in a position to feel adequately advised. The Working Group did

---

[60] WG on EPR Report, Page 39

[61] WG on EPR, page 39, section 4.42

[62] WG on EPR, page 39 section 4.44

however recommend that the Department of Health in England and the devolved administrations carry out further work, in conjunction with stakeholder groups, on the feasibility, costs, and legislative and legal implications and benefits of a licensing regime for health care workers.

The basic benefits offered to the public, by this form of regulation, would theoretically be:-

People receiving services from a licensed worker would know that the worker:

* *had undergone criminal record checks and checks that confirmed that he/she was not on any list of people considered unsuitable to work with vulnerable adults or children;*

* *had undertaken a basic level of training/qualifications (possibly based on standards agreed by Skills for Health); was signed up to a code of conduct and that a means of redress existed if that person breached the relevant code.*

This, however, still does not resolve the problem about what constitutes the appropriate level of training, for the practitioner and for the protection of the continued existence of individual traditions.

In addition, the Working Group recommended that it should also consider whether other professional and occupational groups should be judged to need further regulation.[63]

Despite these reservations, this model was offered as a fully viable option in the consultation document, with the slightly more Draconian version "Statutory Licensing Schemes" receiving an enthusiastic review.

This situation would therefore propose that the Herbal practitioner would be required to rest his/her head under a "sword of Damocles" of unknown size, of unknown weight, of unknown sharpness and suspended by a cord of unspecified tensile strength!

---

[63] WG on EPR, page 40, section 4.45

It was proposed that "Licensing" would control the use of "protected title". This would make it a criminal offence for an unlicensed practitioner to use the protected title with intent to deceive the public. '

This would of course *not* prevent the practitioner undertaking exactly the same therapy under a different title. If Licensing could provide an accepted standard of criminal record check, it would resolve the current situation where an individual has to undergo the expense of repeated checks in a number of situations.
This model of regulation might provide some benefit, once the other questions have been answered and their associated problems resolved.

Statutory Regulation

The theoretical option of Statutory Regulation is one that has been debated with equal amounts of passion, ignorance and misinformation.

The Statutory Regulation of Herbal Medicine has been recommended by the Registrar of the Health Professionals' Council (HPC).

Under the proposals for Statutory Regulation, the title Medical Herbalist would become "protected". It has been proposed that in order to qualify to use the "protected title" of Medical Herbalist, the practitioner would have to have completed a university degree course, approved by either the EHTPA or NIMH: although up to now, several university courses fitting this description have been available, several of these have now collapsed through lack of support.

The theoretical benefits that would be bestowed by Statutory Regulation are that it would guarantee a basic level of training of the therapist, while at the same time providing a level of legal protection to the public against criminal or negligent behaviour.

A certain degree of misinformation has been circulated, indicating that Statutory Regulation by the Health Professionals Council would provide some degree of formal recognition of the profession, leading to (or assisting) its integration within the National Health Service.

There has also been a secondary area of interest, which although only being partially relevant, has been promoted to a level of disproportionate importance.

In 2011 we have been promised (or threatened) with the implementation of The European Directive on Traditional Herbal Medicine Products (THMPD). Concern has been expressed that this will have an impact on the availability of un-licensed herbal medicine, although even this unfounded fear has been challenged by the MHRA.

Section 12(1) herbalists can continue to access unlicensed herbal medicines from their UK suppliers whether SR is implemented or not.[64.]

The proposed restrictions would apply to manufactured products which currently come under the exemptions contained in the section 12 (2) of the current Medicine Act.

This is a separate issue to the availability of Herbal medicines currently available to practitioners under section 12 (1) of the 1968 Medicines Act, relating to herbal medicine provided by the therapist to the patient directly, after a face-to-face consultation.

The implementation of THMPD will continue to allow practitioners to purchase stock from the suppliers and blend prescriptions themselves, without having to be statutorily regulated or hold a manufacturers licence for the finished prescription. This has been confirmed by the MHRA.[65]

The licensing of manufactured products runs to approximately £40,000 per product in development costs. Although a fast track licensing scheme has been implemented for the benefit of herbal products with an established history of safe use, as of yet very few products (reported as being as few as 10) have completed the process. This has created a problem for the manufacturers of these products, some of whom may also be running a prescription service, compiling custom made blends of herbal remedies.

---

[64] Richard Woodfield (MHRA) e-mail dated 6.11.2009

[65] Richard Woodfield (MHRA) e-mail dated 6.11.2009

In the past this has removed the necessity of maintaining "stock" by the practitioner.

It has been proposed that statutory regulated practitioners would be able to continue to commission "third party manufactured" unlicensed products, and prescribe them to their patients. This would of course offer the only available market outlet to the manufacturers of unlicensed herbal medicine products, which otherwise would not exist without the Statutory Regulation of the practitioner.

Unfortunately this argument has been proved to be a fundamentally flawed. The MHRA has confirmed that Statutory Regulation, on its own, will not give the regulated practitioner access to unlicensed "third party" manufactured herbal products. To achieve this, a derogation under Article 5.1 of Directive 2001/83/EC would have to be established, and at present there is no prospect of this happening.

"Derogation" is not, in all probability, a term with which the majority of Herbalists will be familiar. The legal definition is given as being –

"The partial abrogation of a law. To derogate from a law is to enact something which is contrary to it, while to abrogate a law is to abolish it entirely."

In this particular instance, a suitable derogation under Article 5.1 of Directive 2001/83/EC would theoretically allow Herbalists to continue to have access to unlicensed manufactured herbal products and third party prepared prescriptions, in line with previous practice. However, to achieve this, Herbalists would need to become legally categorised as "authorised health-care professionals," with the authority to bypass the legal restrictions (the derogation), which would otherwise prevent this.

Derogation would require a further round of consultations before the enactment of any such legal instrument could be considered. According to the MHRA, there are, at present, no plans to undertake any such consultation process and no anticipation that such a process will be entered into in the foreseeable future.

It does however remain probable that in order to become "authorised health care professionals," Herbalists would have to become statutorily regulated.

Without the enactment of the necessary derogation however, they would only become subject to the associated expenses and restrictions, but without the benefit that they had hoped to achieve. Those, who have vociferously campaigned for the implementation of Statutory Regulation, do not (through their arguments) appear to have been aware of the inefficacy of this proposition.

The British Herb Society, as an association of herbal product manufacturers has been highly in favour of the Statutory Regulation of Herbal practitioners, whether practitioners want it or not. It should be noted however, that the financial benefit to the manufacturers of herbal medicine products is not a valid reason for the Statutory Regulation of herbal practitioners.

Although the supporters of Statutory Regulation previously maintained the stance that its implementation was inevitable, the tone of the more recent WG on EPR reports have called this into question, and have confirmed that the Department of Health is well aware that specific interest groups have attempted to manipulate the regulatory process by making false or exaggerated claims about the alleged dangers to the public associated with various "aspirant" professions.[66]

This has caused considerable concerns about the economic return on investment outlay by the manufacturers of these products, as it would naturally affect their ability to market them. However, as stated earlier in this publication, this is a completely separate issue to the regulatory status of Herbalists, although an extraordinary amount of effort has gone into confusing these two separate issues.

Any benefit that Statutory Regulation might have been claimed to bestow in this area, would be illusory in any case, as the volume of sales through statutorily regulated practitioners would be unlikely to replace that currently available through "over-the-counter" merchandising. In spite of

---

[66] WG on EPR report 16.7.2009 page 43.

this, the staff of the major providers of herbal medicine supplies were photographed vociferously campaigning for the Statutory Regulation of Medical Herbalists outside the House of Commons in November 2009.[67]

In response to the perceived threat posed by the introduction of THMPD, and the recommendation that an appropriate level of regulation for Herbal Medicine should be found, a strange and wondrous dance of confusion was entered into. A steering group was set up for the purposes of making recommendations to Government. One of the major contributors to the steering group was the Chairman of the EHTPA who sat as a "stakeholder" member. As a "stakeholder chair", his authority within the committee was that given to him as a representative of the interests of Herbal Medicine as laid down in the EHTPA constitution.

This has already been quoted as being:-

"The arts and sciences of any and all traditional or complementary systems of medicine (including but not limited to Traditional Chinese Medicine, Western Herbal Medicine, Ayurvedic Medicine and Traditional Tibetan medicine) and in which systems of medicine a main means of treatment is the provision of herbal medicines. It is acknowledged that the definition of what constitutes herbal medicine may vary between traditions and will reflect the legal position as laid down by the UK and EU medicines law and CITES".[68]

As the EHTPA Chairman was there by virtue of that position, it was this position that gave him the alleged authority to represent the interests of Herbal Medicine.

The EHTPA is in effect an umbrella group that draws its authority from the Professional Associations (PAs) that make up its membership.

---

[67] Photograph published on the front page of "Millefolium" the newsletter of Proline Botanicles.

[68] Report to Ministers from The Department of Health Steering Group on the Statutory Regulation of Practitioners of Acupuncture, Herbal Medicine, Traditional Chinese Medicine and Other Traditional Medicine Systems Practised in the UK,

As stated earlier, the original policy of the EHTPA was to promote the Statutory Self-Regulation of Herbal Medicine, as the "least worst" alternative to Voluntary Self Regulation, for the specific purpose of avoiding the imposition of Statutory Regulation.

It was from this position that it had recruited its membership. It is therefore reasonable to suggest that support for Voluntary Self Regulation was part of the mandate its Chairman held, in representing the interests of Herbal Medicine to Government.

This was the limit of the mandate in force on the date of publication of the Steering Group Report in May 2008.
It was not until November 2008 that a vote was taken in one of the larger, or possibly even the largest, PA represented in the EHTPA, the National Institute of Medical Herbalists (NIMH). The purpose of the vote was to seek approval to change the policy of NIMH, in relation to the future regulation of Herbal Medicine.

In the light of the small amount of clear information on the subject available at that time, 68% of the membership felt insufficiently informed to cast a vote either for or against this motion. A mere 28% voted in favour, with the remainder resolutely voting against the proposition.
Although this hardly constituted a majority decision, it was still taken as the mandate to change the official policy of NIMH on this subject.

Until November 2008, when this change took place, the mandated policy had been a preference for Statutory Self Regulation (SSR). It is important to bear this date in mind. As the term "Herbal Medicine" in the context of the Steering Group Report is restricted to the meaning of "Western Herbal Medicine", without reference to the word "traditional", it would be appropriate to examine the stance of the other Professional Associations within the EHTPA allocated to that block.

The Association of Master Herbalists maintain a philosophy that there should be "an herbalist in every home, and a practitioner in every town", and advocates this on the front page of their website.

Such a policy is not commensurate with the belief that the practice of Herbal Medicine is so dangerous that it should be restricted only to those practitioners subject to the most draconian form of regulation available. It also follows a philosophy that it is more important to study the nature of the individual rather than that of the ailment he manifests, before attempting to provide a remedy for the disease.

This mirrors the ancient and honourable tradition advocated as long ago as the time of Hippocrates, who recommended exactly this approach. In spite of this philosophical stance the Association of Master Herbalists professes support for Statutory Regulation.

This pre-Cartesian philosophy stands in stark contrast to that of modern allopathic medicine with which it would make an uncomfortable bedfellow, despite the pro-SR propaganda that Statutory Regulation would elevate the standing of herbal medicine to such a degree that it could be integrated into the health service alongside allopathic practice.

In order to promote this Halcyon ideal, the pro-SR protagonists have attempted to portray Herbal Medicine to be in need of regulation, not because of its efficacy, but on account of the exaggerated claims of danger that they have made on its behalf. The proposal that has therefore been put forward is that the NHS should take up the use of a form of medicine that its own practitioners have branded as dangerous.

The logic of this proposition has yet to be explained by either the Association of Master Herbalists, or any other Professional Associations advocating SR.

The College of Practitioners of Phytotherapy pronounces itself to be wholly in favour of Statutory Regulation, but does so, in part, on the claim that if it were to go ahead-

"Doctors and other health professionals will gain important new partners in helping integrate the healthcare of the 50% of their patients who use herbal remedies."[69]

This advice is in direct contradiction to a statement by the Department of Health, that Statutory Regulation by the HPC does not in any way confer acceptance by the NHS.[70] There is no link between the Statutory Regulation of Herbal practitioners and their ability to work in partnership with "doctors and other health professionals".
In addition to this false assumption, the CPP also states that in the absence of Statutory Regulation-

"The public will forever lose important professional expertise in ensuring standards in their use of herbal remedies and integration with their wider healthcare needs."

As the current level of excellence has been attained without Statutory Regulation, it is difficult to substantiate the claim that an extension of the current status quo will lead to a loss of the existing "professional expertise".

It should also be remembered that Statutory Regulation is only one of a wide range of proposals currently under consideration.

From this, it immediately becomes apparent that yet again the arguments in favour of Statutory Regulation are not only invalid, but irrelevant.

In the light of the current level of expertise and professional standards, of which the College of Practitioners of Phytotherapy is justly proud, this organisation stands as a shining example of the efficacy of Voluntary Self-Regulation, under which it has practised up to now. In the process of demonstrating these high standards, it has undermined the case for the alleged benefits of Statutory Regulation.

---

[69] Extract from PDF file downloaded from College of Practitioners of Phytotherapy website.

[70] Letter from Kate Roy, Customer Service Centre Dept. of Health 16.12.2008

Members of the **Unified Register of Herbal Practitioners** (URHP) have been "whipped" into line, for the purposes of pursuing Statutory Regulation, under the threat of expulsion from their professional Register if they oppose the proposition[71].

This has made it difficult to differentiate between those who genuinely support this measure, and those who opposed it, but feel themselves deprived of their democratic right to dissent.

In addition to this, it would be appropriate to recognize that this organisation is a Register of practitioners of a number of diverse practices that are variously modern, traditional, occidental and oriental.

Under Voluntary Self-Regulation the URHP has been able to monitor and maintain the standards of excellence of its members. In the event of Statutory Regulation coming into force, this organisation would be likely to encounter some difficulties irrespective of the recommendations in the Steering Group Report.

If the Register of practitioners were to be regulated by the Health Professionals Council, it would have to comply with the criteria laid down by the HPC.

Amongst these is the requirement that the Register should practice "a discreet area of activity displaying some homogeneity".

This would immediately present a major problem, as some of the traditions in Herbal Medicine practised by its membership, have not been recommended for Statutory Regulation.

This would lead to a paradoxical and anomalous situation, which would cause the HPC to be in breach of its own constitution should it to attempt to regulate practitioners not covered by Statutory Regulation. In effect, Statutory Regulation would endanger the future existence of the URHP even in its current form; as in becoming statutory regulated, it would be

---

[71] E-mail Sent: Tue, 14 Apr 2009 10:21> Subject: FW: [ukherbal-list] 'Herbal Medicine' petition

consigning itself to history (although this would require the HPC to breach its own constitution).

As the URHP not only shut down its members' forum, but also removed the relevant documentation appertaining to Statutory Regulation from member's area of its website, it is difficult to ascertain how well-informed its members were on this subject.

This possible absence of accurate information might possibly be reflected in the official URHP response to the public consultation document, which on 14 occasions stated that the URHP response was in agreement with the EHTPA response, without actually stating what the EHTPA response was.

A pre-formatted postcard was made available for download from the URHP website, as a public response to the Public Consultation Document. The pre-formatted text stated that the Public Consultation Document had been too complicated to use:-

"I could not fill in the Consultation response online due to its complexity and difficulty of use"

Despite the declared inability to comprehend the issues, the pre-formatted postcard was happy to advocate with complete certainty that:-

"As consumer, I want the Government to establish Statutory

Regulation for Herbal Medicine, Acupuncture, TCM and other traditional medicine systems.

No other arrangement than Statutory Regulation will meet my needs."

On the evidence available, it would be easy to conclude that decision-making without comprehension of or even access to the relevant information is the policy of this organisation. When added to the threat that had already been given to those who dissent from the official line, it questions whether the mandate from the members was democratic and based on unbiased presentation or relevant facts.

Members of the **International Register of Consultant Herbalists and Homoeopaths** (IRCH), which at that time was still a member of the EHTPA, had never even been offered a vote on this change of policy. The IRCH eventually resigned from the EHTPA, because it thought this change in policy was positively detrimental to the future interests of traditional Herbal Medicine.

There was therefore no basis to support any claim that the majority of the members of the Professional Associations within the EHTPA, practising "Herbal Medicine" was actually in favour of Statutory Regulation.

The Steering Group Report supporting the introduction of Statutory Regulation was published in <u>May 2008</u>.

This date is clearly printed on the front cover of the "Report to Ministers from The Department of Health Steering Group on the Statutory Regulation of Practitioners of Acupuncture, Herbal Medicine, Traditional Chinese Medicine and Other Traditional Medicine Systems Practised in the UK", which is available in the public domain.

In <u>May 2008</u> a letter between the EHTPA Chairman and the then Minister of State for Health (Mr Ben Bradshaw) was posted on the EHTPA website. In this letter (dated 7.5.2008), the EHTPA Chairman stated that the EHTPA stakeholder (i.e. himself) had been a major stakeholder in the formulation of the Report by the Steering Group.

The Report had been on the subject of the introduction of Statutory Regulation.

But remember, the EHTPA Chairman did not hold a clear mandate on behalf of Herbal Medicine, although he did claim that the EHTPA represented "some 1,500 practitioners of herbal / traditional medicine across the United Kingdom."

In this there appeared to be some disparity between the accumulated membership of the Professional Associations, and the representation of the views of the majority of the individual members.

Although this might appear to be a matter of mathematical semantics, it becomes one of crucial importance, in gauging any claim for genuine democratic support for Statutory Regulation amongst the profession.

From this it would appear that the EHTPA Chairman might have been promoting a position for which he did not have an authoritative mandate, and therefore only representing a minority opinion.

As the EHTPA Chairman claimed to be a "major stakeholder" in the formulation of the Report, this calls into question the validity of the EHTPA recommendations.

This is an extremely important point, as it has been inferred that:-

a. That there had been enthusiastic voluntary support for Statutory Regulation from the bulk of the membership of the Professional Associations the EHTPA.

b. Without Statutory Regulation, the future of practice of Herbal Medicine would become severely restricted through lack of access to herbal supplies.

Both of these statements have now been demonstrated to be highly questionable.

The question that seems to have been posed is "**If** we can no longer have Voluntary Self-Regulation, and were forced to adopt Statutory Regulation, in order to maintain access to unlicensed manufactured products (even though commercially manufactured products are not part of genuine traditional practice) how would we set about it?"

Even this question has been shown to be inappropriate, as it failed to take into account the lack of the availability of the appropriate derogation under Article 5.1 of Directive 2001/83/EC.

The argument for the alleged necessity for such regulation has centred round a desire to circumvent EU regulations, which concern the safety and licensing of concentrated biochemical manufactured products, rather than finding the appropriate level of regulation for genuine traditional practice.

This disparity, and its associated conflict of interests, has distorted the debate throughout the proceedings.

Access to the appropriate correspondence has revealed that the Report to Ministers from The Department of Health Steering Group on the Statutory Regulation of Practitioners of Acupuncture, Herbal Medicine, Traditional Chinese Medicine and Other Traditional Medicine Systems Practised in the UK has a on more than one occasion been described as "not fit for purpose, as a briefing document for a Minister of her Majesty's Government," although an alternative use was suggested.

It is just possible that the Department of Health also had certain reservations about this document, as it was subsequently sent back to the Working Group on Extending Professional Regulation for further examination and consideration before its proposals were submitted to a public consultation. It therefore becomes apparent that the arguments for Statutory Regulation have been based on a false premise.

A sufficient democratic mandate for the proposition has never been established, and the appropriate criteria for Statutory Regulation have not been met.

***

6

The Benefits of Statutory Regulation
Fact or Myth

Regulated therapists are safe therapists.

The confidence and trust in health care professionals, allegedly assured by BMA regulation, enabled Dr Harold Shipman to become the most prolific serial killer on record. Here the mantra of public protection is again shown to be a complete red herring and totally irrelevant to the true intention behind the driving force behind Statutory Regulation which is the protection of the system itself.

Nurse Beverley Allit (RCN regulated) murdered a number of young babies in her care.

Between them, these two paragons of regulated professions murdered their patients in their homes, murdered their patients in the surgery and murdered their patients on the hospital ward.

Statutory Regulation provides a vehicle for peer group monitoring to maintain professional standards and patient safety.

This is of course is a total contradiction to the experience of Nurse Margaret Haywood, whose efforts to protect the vulnerable and elderly from neglect and abuse, not only failed to achieve that end, but, because she had exposed the failings of her peers, brought about her own expulsion from the nursing profession. Although she was working in an already regulated profession, the benefit that this gave to the public was totally nonexistent.

In spite of a much trumpeted "whistleblower's code" to protect those exposing malpractice for the benefit of the public, she was ruthlessly crucified, and thrown out of the profession she loved for the "crime" of exposing wholesale abuse within the system.

To be within the system is to be vulnerable to the charge of bringing it into disrepute, without reference to the fact that it may already be totally disreputable!

Here it should also be remembered that the murderous activities of Dr Shipman were not called into question by his fellow medical practitioners, but by an **undertaker!**

Statutory Regulation confers official status on regulated therapies making them available to the public on the NHS

Yet another myth! Statutory Regulation does not offer entry into the NHS. This has been confirmed by direct consultation with the National Institute for Clinical Excellence (NICE). It is already the case that the treatments offered by the NHS are at the discretion of the local authorities. This situation would not be changed by Statutory Regulation.

It is already the case that Acupuncture, although still not at present subject to Statutory Regulation, has been available within the National Health Service for a number of years.

Regulated therapies are safe therapies

Of around 2500 [commonly used NHS] treatments covered 13% are rated as beneficial, 23% likely to be beneficial, 8% as trade off between benefits and harms, 6% unlikely to be beneficial, 4% likely to be ineffective or harmful, and 46%, the largest proportion, as unknown effectiveness.[72]

---

[72] BMJ Evidence Centre

It has been admitted that in the decade up to the year 2007, 80,000 patients died from iatrogenic disease and that a further £46 million had been spent by the NHS treating the survivors. Since that time, reports have shown that this state of affairs has further deteriorated; in part blaming the use of increasingly complex MHRA approved drug regimes.

By comparison, those therapies now being attacked with the threat of Draconian regulation are statistically becoming ever increasingly safer! This somewhat makes a mockery of any argument based on these claimed "benefits".

Statutory Regulation will be compulsorily imposed

Sorry, but this is another piece of misinformation put forward by those with a vested interest in abolishing traditional practice in favour of one based predominantly on expensive industrially produced products.

a. Professions need to apply for Statutory Regulation.

b. The level of regulation will be dependent upon the level of threat posed by the therapy.

c. The level of threat should be independently assessed on the same basis as insurance actuary tables, not on grounds of the misleading propaganda being currently circulated, the purpose of which is to bring Herbal Medicine into disrepute in an attempt to get regulation forced upon it.

d. The appropriate mechanisms for evaluating the efficacy of Herbal Medicine, within the framework of Statutory Regulation, do not yet even exist.

You will not be able to practice if you're not Statutory Regulated

Statutory Regulation only gives protection of "title". There is already a whole host of "Osteopaths" opposed to Statutory Regulation, who merely operates under an alternative title.

This is yet another scare story promoted by the pro-Statutory Regulation lobby which has no foundation in fact. The Government is currently studying a raft of proposals for various types of regulation, of which Statutory Regulation is only one proposed option. Regulation by "protected title" would not in any case prevent the "function" of Herbal Medicine being carried out under an alternative "title".

Non-regulated herbalists will not have access to herbs

This is yet another case of misinformation, designed to frighten therapists into voting for an option contrary to their own interests and those of the public.

The only threatened restriction relates to the availability of unlicensed third-party- manufactured herbal products and possibly herbs currently coming under section 12(3) of the current Medicines Act. The possible restrictions do not relate to the herb itself nor prescriptions prepared by the herbalist him/her self.

This is yet another example of the attempt to confuse the regulation of the therapist with the licensing of manufactured products.

The possibility of regulating herbs, outside the format of manufactured products, was discussed and dismissed in the Pittilo Steering Group Report.

11. Pharmacy and Herbal Medicine Practice

It should be noted that there was some discussion as to whether practitioners preparing and supplying unlicensed herbal medicines to meet the needs of individual patients might be statutorily regulated alongside pharmacists.

Little enthusiasm for this option could be identified amongst both pharmacists and herbalists suggesting that such an arrangement could only be achieved by a level of coercion.

As the White Paper determined that the HPC should be the preferred regulator, and in view of other doubts which some members of the

Steering Group had about the appropriateness of this option, we did not pursue the idea further.[73]

There is no connection between the regulation of Herbal practitioners and the implementation of the Traditional Herbal Medicinal Products Directive, as confirmed by an EU document.[74]

"....it should be emphasised that Community legislation on medicinal products, in particular Directive 2001/83/EC laying down the procedures for placing products on the market, follows a product-specific approach and does not attempt to provide a framework for the regulation of traditions of medical practice".

This goes out of its way to make it clear that the THMPD is a piece of legislation connected specifically with herbal products, and unconnected to the regulation of herbal practice / herbal practitioners.[75]

Statutory Regulation would be good for business

Sorry, wrong again! In the event of Statutory Regulation, any one undertaking a regulated therapy under protected title would be limited to the approved parameters of the regulated therapy.

Each regulated therapy in practice would require its own regulatory administration fee, which would eventually have to be paid for out of patients' fees. This would make Herbal Medicine more expensive and therefore less accessible to the public, and would consequently be bad for business.

A similar drastic increase in costs would inevitably be inflicted on a practice based on the use of licensed third party manufactured products the price of which will inevitably rise to recover the cost of implementing THMPD.

---

[73] Page 12 the Steering Group Report to Ministers...

[74] Communication from the Commission to the Council and the European Parliament", dated 29/9/2008, concerning Directive 2001/83/EC as amended by Directive 2004/24/EC, on specific provisions applicable to traditional herbal medicinal products:

[75] Information provided by the Alliance of Natural Health

Between these twin financial pressures the "business" agenda would be best fulfilled by the practitioner remaining (where possible) under Voluntary Self-Regulation, as at present, and restricting his practice to those areas currently allowed under section 12.1 of the 1968 Medicines Act, in the traditional manner.

In the WG on EPR Report it was investigated whether it would be practical for a therapist who was regulated under one title, to practise another regulated therapy under reciprocal arrangements. It was however considered that such a proposal would become too complicated, and therefore too expensive to administer.

The Report does however seem to have created an anomaly within this recommendation. It discussed the possibility of Acupuncture being regulated under its own protected title.
The argument for the Statutory Regulation of Acupuncture was based on the premise of the level of risk posed to the public by a fully qualified practitioner. At the same time it proposed that doctors and nurses, who although qualified in their own professions, but only superficially trained in Acupuncture, would be safe to practise it. This recommendation suggests that the more fully trained you are, the greater the risk you pose to the public. This makes a mockery of the proposed requirement for higher standards of training for the purpose of public safety.

This further poses the question as to whether, or not, the true purpose of Statutory Regulation is the protection of the monopoly of the regulatory process (and its organs), in this case the HPC.

The author of this document had already brought this paradox to the attention of the Department of Health. The Department reiterated the recommendation, but failed to produce an explanation to resolve the anomaly. It did however confirm that a therapy only had to be approved, and not statutorily regulated, to be used in the NHS.
This further established that SR is completely irrelevant, as far as this issue is concerned.

Statutory Regulation protects the public's freedom of choice

As Statutory Regulation imposes a closed shop based on a one size fits all paradigm of training, the variety of traditions and approaches of therapeutic practice become automatically curtailed.
As already demonstrated, the very existence of Traditional Western Herbal Medicine has already been set to become institutionally denied within the Steering Group Report, upon which the subsequent WG on EPR reports and the public consultation document were based.

Statutory Regulation will protect the traditions through protected title.

Although it is stated in the HPC website that regulation would protect the traditions, it would have exactly the opposite effect, by effectively forcing them to comply with one approved model of training.

The "one size fits all" officially imposed paradigm of training is totally incompatible with the maintenance of the diverse traditions, and would lead to the loss of the 5000 year old canon of empirical knowledge enshrined in traditional medicine.

***

7

MHRA and Herbal Medicine

The MHRA and the Pharmaceutical Industry

The THMPD gives control of licensed and unlicensed herbal medicines to the MHRA, a medicines regulator that is entirely funded by fees from the pharmaceutical industry. A House of Commons Health Committee Report from 2005, entitled 'The Influence of the Pharmaceutical Industry' is highly critical of the MHRA and its close relationship with the pharmaceutical industry. It states:- '(t)here are regular interchanges of staff, common policy objectives, agreed processes, shared perspectives and routine contact and consultation. Many of the senior staff of the MHRA have previously worked with the industry ...' It is therefore doubtful whether the MHRA can be trusted to serve the best interests of herbal medicines, herbalists and their patients. [76]

This extract of a report from the House of Commons Health Committee, can be downloaded from the web address below, and is highly critical of the way the MHRA regulates the pharmaceutical industry. [77]

It goes on to state:-

"The consequences of lax oversight are that the industry's influence has expanded and a number of practices have developed which act against the public interest," ....

---

[76] Quote from Herbal Medicine and the Law – A Critique

[7] http://www.publications.parliament.uk/pa/cm200405/cmselect/cmhealth/42/42.pdf

"The Department of Health has not only to promote the interests of the pharmaceutical industry but also the health of the public and the effectiveness of the NHS. There is a dilemma here which cannot be readily glossed over. The Secretary of State for Health cannot serve two masters. The department seems unable to prioritise the interests of patients and public health over the interests of the pharmaceutical industry. We therefore recommend that sponsorship of the industry pass from the department of Health to the Department of Trade and Industry."[78]

From this it becomes clear that the House of Commons Committee not only believed that the MHRA was antipathetic to the interests of Herbal Medicine, but had already been putting the business interests of the pharmaceutical companies before the health interests of the public! It is difficult to understand why any Herbalist should wish to become embroiled in such a dysfunctional regime, and effectively give it control of his or her profession.

Questions also arise about why an organisation such as the EHTPA, that is constitutionally bound to protect and promote the interests of Herbal Medicine, should align itself with the arguments and policies of an organisation officially antipathetic to the interests of Herbal Medicine, its practitioners and their patients.

Any move to bring traditional Herbal Medicine deeper into the zone of influence of the MHRA, would therefore be contrary to the interests of the practitioner and patient and could only be of benefit to the pharmaceutical companies through their ability to influence the erosion of availability of herbal products.

This has proved to be a major problem in India, where Government has had to take active steps to protect herbal medicines from "bio prospecting" by the pharmaceutical companies, seeking to patent the use of certain herbs or herbal extracts and thereby claim them as their own. This was reported on at some length by Randeep Ramesh in the Guardian newspaper on the 22nd of

---

[78] A House of Commons Health Committee Report from 2005, entitled 'The Influence of the Pharmaceutical Industry'

February 2009 in an article titled "India moves to protect traditional medicines from foreign patents"

Within the greater context, it might be appropriate to consider the manufacturers of herbal-based medicinal compounds as pharmaceutical companies, in that the manufacture of standardised extracts provides concentrated extraction of biochemical elements in a form that does not occur in nature and without reference to those parts of the plant discarded in the process. This practice has only served to confuse the boundaries between natural medicine and a model based on pharmaceutical products.

The human organism never encountered any such substances during its evolution, and may therefore potentially experience difficulty in processing material of this nature.

These products might therefore be regarded as Frankensteinian pharmaceuticalized preparations that should not in any way be compared with those used in Traditional Herbal Medicine.
There is a danger that any problems arising from the use of these unnatural products, might be used to tarnish the record of natural herbal medicines, and effectively be used as a stick with which to beat it.

This has already happened in the case of Kava-kava, a root now banned in concentrated dry extract and in the more dilute tincture used by traditional Herbalists and even water extracts (infusions) as used in the Polynesian islands, its place of origin, (where it is still available).

It is a matter of interest that the obsessive protagonists of the unsubstantiated requirement for the implementation of Statutory Regulation, have often quoted the views of the MHRA that these unnatural concentrated (although) herb-based pharmaceutical preparations have the potential to interact with allopathic drugs.

Although the MHRA may have some justification with this concern, the same problem does not arise with the traditional use of herbal tinctures, decoctions or infusions, which can be used safely. This highlights one of the essential differences between a practise based on Traditional Herbal Medicine and one founded primarily on the use of highly concentrated standardised extracts, and it remains essential that this differentiation be maintained under the future regulation of Herbal Medicine.

A high degree of confusion amongst Herbalists, about how statutory regulated status would affect their ability access to manufactured products has muddied the waters of debate on the subject of regulation of the practitioner.

The position on this, as stated by the MHRA is:-

"Fiction: Unless SR is implemented by 2011, section 12(1) herbalists would be unable to access a wide range of 'manufactured' herbal medicines.

Fact: In 2011, 'manufactured' herbal medicines will come within the scope of the Traditional Herbal Medicinal Products Directive (THMPD) and will continue to be available to herbalists regardless whether SR is implemented or not."[79]

It should be noted that this statement does not differentiate between licensed and unlicensed manufactured products. So, although this statement might be strictly accurate, it might also prove misleading to the naive reader. It will only be <u>licensed</u> manufactured herbal medicines that will continue to be available to herbalists regardless whether or not SR is implemented.

Realistically, it might be improbable to suppose that an unlicensed product only available through regulated herbalists would have an economically sustainable market, even if the necessary derogation were implemented to allow this to come about.

The Statutory Regulation of the Herbalist would not put a single unlicensed product back onto the shelves for the over-the-counter market. The argument that the Statutory Regulation of the Practitioner would in any way maintain the availability of unlicensed manufactured products, might therefore be seen as a complete red herring.

---

[79] Richard Woodfield (MHRA) 6.11.2009

This however has not prevented a number of organisations from promoting this alleged benefit in support of their argument for SR.

The MHRA has confirmed that unlicensed manufactured products will not be available to the public, the unregulated practitioner or to the statutorily regulated practitioner, under any circumstances currently applying under UK law.

As it would take some time to undertake the necessary consultations and enact the required legal instruments to bring the necessary derogation into effect, the manufacturers of unlicensed herbal products would have to spend an indefinite interlude without being able to undertake any trade in their products. It is difficult to imagine the continued financial viability of any such situation.

The pragmatic resolution to the situation could only lie in their return to becoming wholly dependent on trading in a form of Herbal Medicine not dependent on licensing, unless they are both able and prepared to fund the licensing process of a substantial range of manufactured products, in the hope that the market will sustain the costs that this would inevitably entail.

Many of the problems faced by the manufacturers of herbal products, have been brought about by the reinterpretation of the terminology relating to them.

This reinterpretation of what constitutes a "manufactured" product was introduced to facilitate the introduction of THMPD.

As this problem has been brought about by an exercise in creative semantics, it is quite possible that the manufacturing companies will seek to avoid at least some of the restrictions of THMPD, by investigating other criteria for marketing their products.

Although such manoeuvres might maintain some of the current availability of herbal preparations, this still remains a separate issue to the search for the appropriate form of regulation of Medical Herbalists, in accordance to the level of risk posed by the individual traditions.

***

8

Public consultation

It is understood from copies of correspondence posted on the EHTPA website, that there had been an expectation on the part of the EHTPA Chairman for the Steering Group Report to be swiftly followed by a public consultation on its contents.

A letter dated **15.1.09** was sent by the Assistant Director of Human Resources to the EHTPA Chairman explaining the delay, and was posted on the EHTPA website. It was also explained in this letter that the Government had decided to refer the matter to the Working Group on Extending Professional Regulation, and would not launch a public consultation until after the findings of the WG on EPR had been considered.

Attention should be given to the date of this letter.

On the **30th of January**, 15 days later, there was a posting on the EHTPA website indicating that the public consultation was expected to commence in February and run until June. An individual, who is not unknown to the author, did not come across this EHTPA posting until May. He had officially been listed as an "interested party" to be notified by the Department of Health on the commencement of the Public Consultation, and had not been so notified; nor was he able to find any trace of the Public Consultation Document on the Department of Health website, he was a little bemused by this apparent contradictory state of affairs.

As this individual could imagine some possible explanations for this paradox, he wrote to the Department of Health for clarification about whether the true state of affairs was either:-

a) A public consultation was actually under way of which the interested party had not been informed, and which was posted on some other than the Department of Health website.

b) There was a phantom Public Consultation allegedly being undertaken, of which the fictional results which would be declared in due course.

c) There was no public consultation taking place, and the EHTPA had intimated at the smooth forward progress of its project, while knowing this not to be the case.

The response from the Department of Health confirmed that at that time, the report was still under consideration by the Working Group on Extending Professional Regulation, and that the Public Consultation would be launched at a later date.

The actual date of the publication of the Public Consultation Document was eventually listed on its cover as being the 1st of June 2009, with it being made publicly available on the 3rd August, with responses to be submitted on-line from the 4th onwards. Its closing date was advertised as being the 2nd of November 2009.

In response to the publication of the Public Consultation Document, there appeared a number of pre-formatted responses proposed by the professional associations under the EHTPA umbrella.

This was put forward as guidance to both their membership and members of the public.

As these pre-formatted responses were prepared by the various professional bodies, the naive reader might conclude that they were the result of thoughtful and informed consideration, and be in line with the consensus of opinion of the memberships involved.

With this in mind, it might be constructive to review these offerings put forward as expert and informed opinion.

In the "authorised" submission from the Unified Register of Herbal Practitioners (URHP), the questions repeatedly offered the following response:-

"We fully endorse the answer and comments made to this question by the EHTPA in its Consultation Document response already submitted to the Department of Health."

This response, and variations of it, were put forward on no less than 14 occasions.

Anyone wishing to pursue the nature of this response would have to enquire at the EHTPA about the nature of the opinion of the URHP, as the URHP had apparently not been up to the task of formulating its own answer.

It would seem therefore that it had been left to the EHTPA to undertake this task on its behalf, thereby being able to rest assured that the URHP response did not go "off message".

It was of course equally possible that the URHP had not been able to understand the questionnaire itself.

On its website, it offered the following preformatted postcard, which it offered to the public along with the recommendation that copies be sent to the Government:-

"Re: DOH Dear Department of Health Response Team, Joint Consultation of the Report to Ministers from the DH Steering Group on the Statutory Regulation of Acupuncture, Herbal Medicine, Traditional Chinese Medicine and Other Traditional Medicine Systems Practised in the UK As consumer, I want the Government to establish Statutory Regulation for Herbal Medicine, Acupuncture, TCM and other traditional medicine systems.

No other arrangement than Statutory Regulation will meet my needs.

I could not fill in the Consultation response online due to its complexity and difficulty of use."

Here URHP seems to be advocating that members of the public should vote for a regulation that they did not understand themselves, and do so on the advice of an organisation unable to present either its own response, or the reasoning upon which that response had been made! Without the availability of the relevant information upon which to base a judgement or recommendation, the concept of informed consent cannot possibly exist; and yet this is exactly the stance of the URHP in relation to the Public Consultation Document!

In the light of the argument above, it is highly questionable whether any alleged support for Statutory Regulation, obtained by this means, actually has any validity! The apparent lack of openness and ability to accept debate amongst its own membership might seem to indicate that the EHTPA response may not necessarily reflect the views of the URHP membership itself.

Any lack of enthusiasm experienced by the members of URHP might be explained by the possibility that they may have been sufficiently diligent to consult the HPC website; and informed themselves about the criteria that the aspirant Register would have to fulfil in order to qualify for HPC regulation.

Aspirant groups must:

o   Cover a discreet area of activity displaying some homogeneity.

o   Apply a defined body of knowledge.

o   Practice based on evidence of efficacy.

o   Have at least one established professional body which accounts for a significant proportion of that occupational group.

o   Have independently assessed entry qualifications.

o   Have standards in relation to conduct, performance and ethics.

o   Fitness to practise procedures to enforce those standards.

o   Be committed to continuous professional development (CPD).[80]

---

[80] HPC Criteria for admission as publicly available on the HPC website.

Although the membership of URHP is comprised of practitioners of the highest ability, the Register itself fails to comply with all the requirements described above.

This shortcoming had not deterred the authors of the Steering Group Report from recommending that the URHP be transferred into the HPC under grandparenting arrangements. It was certainly within the power of the Steering Group to recommend whatever it wanted, but it was not within its gift to actually deliver on those recommendations.

The peddling of promises that cannot be fulfilled as a means of garnering support for a conceptually unsound project, might perhaps be seen as an insult not only to themselves, but also to the many and diverse traditions practised by the members of the Register.

It is, in fact, this very multiplicity of traditions that might have been seen to stand in the way of the HPC ever being able to accept URHP amongst its ranks.

The criterion at the top of the list was the requirement that the Register should:-

"Cover a discreet area of activity displaying some homogeneity."[81]

The URHP cannot reasonably be described as being involved in a "discreet area of activity" since its membership practises a wide range of diverse traditions. Although some of the areas of activity had been recommended for Statutory Regulation, the majority had not. This could have produced an anomalous situation that would have lead to the HPC statutorily regulating therapists of a tradition that had not qualified for Statutory Regulation.

If the Register had purely been one of practitioners of Traditional Chinese Medicine, this criterion would not have presented a problem.

If the Register had purely been one of practitioners of Herbal Medicine (within the limited and erroneous description specified in the report) this criterion would not have been a problem either.

---

[81] HPC Criteria for admission as publicly available on the HPC website

The fact of the matter is that the Register is made up of practitioners of Traditional Chinese Medicine, Traditional Western Herbal Medicine, Ayurvedic Medicine, Traditional Tibetan Medicine, Unani Tibb, Naturopathy, Bio-energetic Assessment, Phylac Spagyrics, Kinesiology, Aromatherapy, Reiki, Hypnotherapy, Indian Head Massage, NAET (allergy elimination), Nutritional Therapy, Radionics, Acupuncture, Iridology, Tui Na, Japanese Acupuncture and Homoeopathy.

Amongst the list of members are those who describe their tradition as being "East/West Herbal College.

This would seem to indicate an interesting and dynamic fusion of cultures that defies the "tick the box" labelling system of the HPC.

Many of their practitioners describe their tradition as being Western Tradition, and this is correct since they gained their training and qualification from the International Register of Consultant Herbalists and Homoeopaths that specialises in the training of <u>Traditional</u> Western Herbal Medicine.

Discrepancies such as this demonstrate how the inherent anomalies in the original Steering Group Report became replicated throughout the later Government reports based upon it.

Other pre-formatted responses to the Public Consultation questionnaire included such gems as:-

"Yes, we agree with the proposals for "grandparenting" in the Pittilo. We feel this is fair to all."[82]

As some of the proposals in the Pittilo report were blatantly discriminatory in their nature (see following comments relating to "grandparenting" criteria 4&5, as proposed in the Pittilo, Steering Group Report), it is difficult to know how they can substantiate this statement.

Two of the criteria for grandparenting, laid down in the Pittilo Steering Group Report, had nothing whatever to do with the subject of the safety or

---

[82] URHP public consultation response, publically available on the URHP website.

proficiency of existing practitioners of Herbal Medicine, traditional or otherwise.

Criterion 4

With regard to accrediting educational programmes, effective procedures should be in place to
(a) approve programmes of study,
(b) monitor over a period of time their effectiveness against the stated aims and objectives for the programmes taking account of the success of students in attaining these stated, intended learning outcomes and
(c) reviewing over time the continuing validity of these aims and objectives.

Criterion 5

There must be an absolute separation between the financial/business activity of the organisation and those responsible for the accreditation and monitoring of educational programmes.
It is acceptable for individuals to act as an accreditor butthey should not stand to gain from a successful outcome.[83]

These criteria clearly demonstrate that regulations, that properly belong to the administration of an accrediting body and a teaching body, were being incorrectly applied to a Register of existing experienced practitioners.

Course accreditation, the delivery of educational courses and the actual practice of Herbal Medicine by a qualified professional practitioner are three completely separate functions that became inappropriately confused in the drafting of these criteria.

This subsequently led to a body of experienced professionals being discriminated against by the misapplication of inappropriate criteria.

---

[83] Page 160 of the Steering Group Report

Confusions such as this have been identified by some as being the signature of the Steering Group Report, which is seen as being little more than a collection of non-sequiturs and paradoxical anomalies. This was one of the many detailed aberrations that were raised with the WG on EPR, prior to the drafting of the Consultation Document. Unfortunately, questions such as this, contained in the Consultation Document, related back to the unreconstructed confusions in the original Steering Group Report.

This became a matter of the utmost concern to one organisation in particular (The International Register of Consultant Herbalists and Homoeopaths) as this Register is associated with one of this country's longest standing faculties teaching Traditional Western Herbal Medicine.

These criteria were amongst those inappropriately used as a vehicle to block a recommendation for grandparenting under the Pittilo report. The traditional model of Herbal Medicine, historically taught and practised by the IRCH, is a philosophically at variance with that of NIMH.

The IRCH's continued existence therefore constitutes a threat to the ability of NIMH to become the sole inheritors of the protected title "Herbal Medicine", as these diversities challenged the requirement laid down in the WG on EPR report that discipline had to be defined before it could be regulated.

The various reports, and the subsequent Public Consultation Document, might therefore be seen as a battleground, not only for philosophical dominance, but continued existence, with the dubious benefits of Statutory Regulation forming the backdrop to the drama.

At the same time, another organisation (The Unified Register of Herbal Practitioners) was recommended for grandparenting, despite a significant number of the members of URHP being graduates of the IRCH, while the members of the IRCH, who had actually taught them their craft, were excluded.

The URHP might perhaps have some difficulty in supporting regulations that would effectively block the future training of one of their own paradigms, while at the same time claiming that the practitioners of the same paradigm, (as long as they were members of URHP) were ready to be regulated by the HPC.

This paradoxical anomaly was seen as the breach of natural justice. Protestations to this effect were made directly to Professor Pittilo, the Chairman of the Steering Group Committee. No response was forthcoming. Similar protestations were made to the Chairman of the EHTPA/stakeholder member of the Steering Committee. No response was forthcoming.

Further representations were made to Professor Pittilo about previous discrimination made on the basis of the Steering Group Report against an aspirant Register, which had not undertaken Criminal Record Bureau (CRB) checks on its members, as had been repeatedly requested by the EHTPA.

Direct consultation with the Criminal Records Bureau (see below) confirmed that, at that time, a voluntary Register of self employed professionals could not legally carry out CRB checks on its members. To discriminate against an individual on this basis, would have involved a criminal offence, i.e. The Misuse of Information under the Data Protection Act. No response was forthcoming.

The response from the CRB, on this subject, had been as follows:-

Thank you for your Email.

Businesses with the owner declared as self-employed by definition signifies they're not in a regulated position and as such eliminates them from using the Disclosure Service.
I understand the reservation you have and this is very commendable, but Disclosures are essentially a tool for making a recruitment decision and here this would not apply.

You have two options you may use:
You could request the practitioners to approach a central Police Station and request a 'subject access request (SAR)' check (not all forces carry-out these checks) - if they agree, the Police will activate a localised background check. This may take up to 20 days and is sent via post. I

must emphasise that this is voluntary; only the individual can make the decision to activate the SAR; <u>under no circumstances can this be used to make a recruitment decision. If you did, you could be prosecuted for the misuse of information under the Data Protection Act.</u>

Please see this link for detailed guidance:
www.crb.qov.uk/default.aspx?page=417

The final and best option in my opinion, would be to apply for a Basic Disclosure via Disclosure Scotland (open to all UK residents with a current UK address);

<u>www.disclosurescotland.co.uk</u> - please use this link for guidance.

I hope this was of assistance.
Kind Regards

Mike Valentine, RB Support Officer, Registration Management Unit, Criminal Records Bureau,

It is generally held that if the fulfilment of regulation (in this case Statutory Regulation) were to require the commission of the criminal offence, that the regulation (in this case Statutory Regulation) would be legally invalid.

Incidentally, what the relevant criteria actually said was:-

10. There should be evidence that the body is aware of the importance of criminal record disclosure and the necessity for this in order to protect the public.[84]

Criminal record disclosure was of course included in the declaration document that was required to be signed by every applicant member and renewable with each annual renewal of membership.

From this it became evident that the assessment process for compliance with the proposed criteria was severely flawed, or perhaps even biased; legally it would have been impossible to reject any Register on this basis.

---

[84] Page 161 of the Steering Group Report

Conversely, if one Register was to be rejected on this basis, so would every other register as well, as none of them would have been able to legally comply with this criterion. Had any of the Registers actually carried out CRB checks on members in order to make recruitment decisions, they would have been committing a criminal offence which would have precluded their adoption by the HPC.

Further representations on this subject were made to the Chairman of the EHTPA/stakeholder member of the steering committee. No response was forthcoming.

These paradoxical anomalies go some way to demonstrate the undemocratic and misinformed thinking that has gone into the proposals put forward in the Steering Group Report, which subsequently formed the basis of the Public Consultation Document.

The URHP pre-formatted response also presented the following disingenuous gem.

"We feel strongly that clear communication, both understanding and speaking, is essential in a consultation or advice situation for the safety of the person seeking the advice or consultation."

This appears be a direct contradiction to its own policy of shutting down its members' forum and preventing open debate on whether the adoption of Statutory Regulation was really such a good idea after all. The irony of this statement appears to have escaped the individual who drafted it.

Of course URHP is by no means the only Register to have pre-formatted a pro-Statutory Regulation response to the Public Consultation document in terms unable to withstand close scrutiny.

The RCHM's draft response to the Department of Health's Consultation Document.

(RCHM= Register Chinese Herbal Medicine)

Question 3 (of the consultation document)

What do you envisage would be the benefits to the public, to practitioners, and to businesses, associated with introducing Statutory Regulation?

"The question that should be asked here is rather what would the loss be to members of the public, to practitioners and to businesses if Statutory Regulation does not go ahead.

If SR is not forthcoming many of our member practitioners, and others in the herbal sector will not be able to practice because they rely on third-party supply of herbal medicines for their patients. The expense of running ones own dispensary is not financially viable.

A knock-on effect of this will be that a great many of our Approved Suppliers (those which have undergone an independent quality assurance audit and are committed to raising standards within the sector) will go out of business because of the loss of such third party supply......."

Although the RCHM response addresses their legitimate concerns, it fails to take into account the information provided by the MHRA, that Statutory Regulation would not provide the remedy for this problem without the necessary derogation under Article 5 in place.

The response is therefore based on a completely false argument about which the RCHM appears to be unaware. These are precisely the sort of considerations that were outlined in the WG on EPR Report as being unacceptable arguments to support Statutory Regulation. It should also be noted that, strictly speaking, the RCHM has opted to answer a different question to the one actually asked.

The actual question was based on the expected benefits of SR being introduced, not problems that were expected to arise if it were not.

Further down the response it states:-

"The upshot is that after 2011, in the absence of Statutory Regulation, there is likely to be a significant reduction in the range of herbal medicines that herbal practitioners can use and a corresponding

reduction in consumer choice. Both practitioners and the public would gain from preserving the existing scope of access to herbal medicinal products".

This however seems to be a direct contradiction to information provided by Mr Richard Woodfield from the MHRA, who might be considered the most appropriate metaphorical "horse's mouth" from which to access reliable information on this subject.

<u>Fiction</u>: *Unless SR is implemented by 2011, section 12(1) of the Medicines Act 1968 will be superseded by the Traditional Herbal Medicinal Products Directive (THMPD) and European medicines legislation, effectively banning the practise of herbal medicine in the UK.*

<u>Fact</u>: *Section 12(1) of the Medicines Act 1968 remains available to herbalists in the UK beyond 2011, whether SR is implemented or not.*

And in addition to this he also stated:-

<u>Fiction</u>: *Unless SR is implemented by 2011, section 12(1) herbalists would not have access to unlicensed herbal medicines. Only Registered/licensed herbal medicines or homemade remedies would be available to their patients.*

<u>Fact</u>: *Section 12(1) herbalists can continue to access unlicensed herbal medicines from their UK suppliers whether SR is implemented or not.*

It would therefore appear that once again the pro-Statutory Regulation Professional Associations of the EHTPA is giving out information that does not stand up to critical analysis. It should however be noted, as stated in previous chapter, that section 12 (1) relates to Herbal Medicine in its basic form, and not after it has been subjected to a manufacturing process under the revised interpretation of the terminology.

The use of "third party" manufactured products might constitute a convenience to the modern practitioner, but as in the case of Traditional Western Herbal Medicine, it might be difficult to make a case to substantiate their use as part of genuine traditional practice. There is a "fast track" for the licensing of herbal medicine products with a proven history of safe use over the past few decades, but such limited time span can hardly be termed "traditional" in relation to a paradigm stretching back 5000 years!

Here again, the Public Consultation Document appears to have become embroiled in a number of issues that lie outside the declared purpose to find the appropriate level of regulation for the profession under consideration, appropriate to the risk posed by its practice.

Question 8 (consultation document)

How might the risk of harm to the public be reduced other than by statutory professional self regulation? For example, by voluntary self-regulation underpinned by consumer protection legislation and by greater public awareness, by accreditation of voluntary registration bodies, or by a statutory or voluntary licensing regime?

In our answer to question 6 above, we have stressed that none of these options is satisfactory and that Statutory Regulation is the only appropriate solution.

Here the RCHM is apparently implying that, without the introduction of Statutory Regulation, the practice of Traditional Chinese medicine represents a danger to the public.

Up until now, the RCHM has continued to maintain the highest standards under the current regime of Voluntary Self-Regulation. There is no reason to suggest that the Register of Chinese Herbal Medicine would allow its outstanding professional standards to deteriorate, if the status quo were to prevail.

At the same time it clearly states on its own website:-

"There is a very real possibility that the Government will <u>not</u> proceed with Statutory Regulation".

From this it would seem that the RCHM would prefer no regulation all, if it cannot have the one that it prefers, even if several of the reasons for this preference are either a direct contravention of the allowable criteria, or would not deliver the desired benefit.

The RCHM has also continued to confirm the problems that relate to the evidence base efficacy, that is a requirement for Statutory Regulation by the HPC.

"We would not dispute that there is much more to be done in this direction (developing an evidence base for herbal medicine), but it is important at the same time not to be mesmerised by the claims of one type of evidence, which may not be appropriate for all types of medical intervention."

Concerns have already been expressed to the Government about the breadth of the public consultation process. As the Public Consultation Document has been published within the labyrinthine structure of the Department of Health website, the majority of the public remained completely unaware of its existence, and many of those, who were aware of it, would have experienced considerable difficulty in locating it. If the public in general have not been able to access the document, it is difficult to maintain the illusion that it has been effectively consulted by this process.

The document itself constitutes a masterpiece of clarity dealing with complex issues in a straightforward and unambiguous way. The one area, where it might deserve some criticism, lies in its presentation of "Licensing" as a currently viable option for regulation.

The presentation does not represent the many unresolved and varying factors described in the WG on EPR report by Dr Livingstone. Without comparing these reports, the public would not be adequately informed about the inherent anomalies in this "option".

Several organisations, with an interest in the implementation of Statutory Regulation, have publicly stated their belief that the document and its subject matter are too difficult to comprehend.

Such a statement might be seen as an insult to the intelligence of any diligent well informed reader, (with an understanding of the subject upon which they were being consulted). The problem lies not with the comprehensibility of the document, but with its accessibility.

The figures quoted in relation to earlier consultations have already demonstrated that their penetration into the public awareness has been extremely shallow. This issue was raised with the Department of Health several months before the launch of the current Public Consultation, and concerns over this issue where indeed included in the WG on EPR final report.

There remains a danger that the constituency of voters on this issue may have been disproportionately limited to those of a narrow vested interest in its outcome. Unless a much wider constituency can be shown to have been effectively consulted on this issue, great care should be taken in interpreting the findings of the consultation.

It has widely been stated that over 50% of the population use Herbal Medicine in one form or another.

This issue therefore directly affects the interests of the majority of the population of this country, and it would subsequently be inappropriate to make radical changes to the accessibility to such a widely supported regime of health care, without first having ascertained a genuine informed democratic support for any such measure.

***

9

Summary

1) Any move to restrict the public from having direct access to medical herbs would constitute an act of cultural and religious discrimination, contrary to existing EU policy on protecting cultural diversity.

2) Voluntary Self-Regulation is a successful pre-existing model.

3) As there is already a pre-existing model, an extremely strong case based on public safety would have to be made to compulsorily supplant it with Statutory Regulation.

4) The proportional level of risk has not been established.

5) Without an unacceptable level of risk having been established, Statutory Regulation needs to be applied for and cannot be imposed.

6) There is no majority support for the Statutory Regulation of Herbal Medicine, traditional or otherwise, amongst its practitioners.

7) The cost of Statutory Regulation has not been justified.

8) Such support for the Statutory Regulation of Herbal Medicine, traditional or otherwise, that has been generated amongst its practitioners, has in part been the result of a campaign of misinformation, intimidation and false promises.

9) Statutory Regulation by the HPC does not constitute approval by the NHS.

10) Therapies approved by the NHS do not have to be statutorily regulated.

11) There is no link between the Statutory Regulation of the practitioner and THMPD.

12) There are a number of options available to provide appropriate levels of regulation, in the public interest, including an extension of the current situation.

13) As of yet, there are no appropriate models for evaluating the efficacy of traditional Herbal Medicine.

14) Without an effective model for evaluating evidence of efficacy, a basic requirement for Statutory Regulation has not been met.

15) The Statutory Regulation of Herbal Medicine would detract from the public's freedom of choice.

16) The Statutory Regulation of Herbal Medicine would endanger and not protect the traditions.

17) The Statutory Regulation of Herbal Medicine could not protect the public from misconduct as demonstrated by Shipman and Allit cases.

18) The Statutory Regulation of Herbal Medicine will not maintain the free availability of over-the-counter unlicensed manufactured herbal medicine products to the public.

19) The Statutory Regulation of Herbal Medicine will not increase the practitioner's access to unlicensed manufactured herbal products on behalf of his patients.

20) Any recommendations of the EHTPA Chairman/steering group stakeholder chair for regulation beyond Statutory Self Regulation, would have been outside his mandate as a representative of the interests of Herbal Medicine, whether traditional or otherwise.

21) The validity of the recommendations in the Steering Group Report has been called into question.

22) With the loss of validity of the Steering Group Report, the validity of all subsequent reports is similarly called into question.

23) The Public Consultation Document cannot be justified as being a genuine public consultation, as the majority of the public has remained unaware of its existence.

24) The Public Consultation Document, as a means of validating any significant change to the provision of Herbal Medicine, whether traditional or otherwise, cannot be supported without the majority of the public having been effectively consulted on such a change.

25) The fitness of the MHRA to act as an unbiased advisor on the safety of Herbal Medicine has been officially called into question.

26) There is an established history of pharmaceutical companies attempting to patent the use of traditional herbal medicines, and remove their free availability to the public.

27) There is a need to maintain the independence of herbal medicines outside the influence and control of pharmaceutical companies and organisations influenced by them.

***

10

Conclusion

The European Union has issued a directive that requires the licensing of herbal medicine manufactured products (THMPD). To enable this directive to come into effect, the MHRA redefined its interpretation of "manufactured products". These products up to now have been available under section 12 (2) of the Medicines Act.

Herbal Medicine that has not been defined as "manufactured product" will continue to be available, as is currently the case, under section 12 (1) of the Medicines Act.

Independent from the incoming licensing requirements for herbal medicine products, the Government has set about a consultation process to evaluate the most appropriate form of regulation that should be applied to practitioners of Medical Herbalism. A number of options are currently being considered, each with its strengths and weaknesses.

The Government has proposed, as a basic ground rule that the degree of regulation should be proportional to the risk posed by the therapy. It has also ruled that the cost of regulation should be proportional to the effective benefit gained by any chosen form of regulation. This stipulation rules out the possibility of applying a disproportionate form of regulation, to guard against extremely rare occurrences.

The EHTPA has promoted the idea that Statutory Regulation would be of benefit to the future interests of Herbal Medicine.

For the purposes of this type of regulation, the various traditions have to be independently assessed to establish their "evidence of efficacy" in order to comply with the requirements of the HPC.

The models for measuring efficacy have only been established in relation to allopathic medicine. As of yet, an appropriate mechanism for establishing "evidence of efficacy" has not been established in relation to traditional Herbal Medicine. In addition, the necessary funds, to establish such a model, are not currently available.

Of all forms of Herbal Medicine that are currently practised in this country, only two have been proposed for Statutory Regulation. The two modalities, for which this degree of regulation has been recommended by the HPC, are Traditional Chinese Medicine and (Western) Herbal Medicine. Within this recommendation, no recognition was made of the unique holistic approach of Traditional Western Herbal Medicine.

The case for regulation has been based on exaggerated claims of dangerous toxicity connected with the components used in the practice of these two paradigms.

A strategy was entered into, that involved bringing Herbal Medicine into sufficient disrepute in an attempt to coerce the Government into imposing Statutory Regulation on Herbal Medicine and TCM.

This was a misguided attempt to increase the professional profile of practitioners of these two disciplines.

The main purpose behind this manoeuvre was an erroneous belief that statutorily regulated practitioners would continue to have access to unlicensed manufactured herbal products after the imposition of the European Herbal Medicine Products Directive (THMPD).

The MHRA has openly declared that, even in the event of Statutory Regulation being brought into force in relation to these two disciplines, they still not would have achieved access to unlicensed manufactured herbal products. For this to come about, these two professions would not only have to be statutorily regulated, but they would also have to have access to a derogation under Article 5.1 of Directive 2001/83/EC, which does not currently exist in Britain.

Even if this strategy has been able to deliver the intended benefits, it would have left a number of other traditions of Herbal Medicine without similar benefit. This would have been highly divisive to the traditions in question, effectively relegating them to second-class status in the public perception.

In order to gain support for this plan, it was widely put forward that Statutory Regulation by the Health Professionals Council would in some way raise the official standing of Herbalists, and bring them within the NHS. This was a complete mis-representation of the facts, as the Department of Health has directly confirmed that regulation does not in any way represent professional recognition by the Health Service.

As the dust settles, we have been left with a situation in which the general public has become indoctrinated with a belief that Herbal Medicine is disproportionately dangerous, and is better avoided in favour of allopathic medicine; despite a large amount of evidence demonstrating the possible lethal consequences of making such a choice. The directors of this strategy are therefore guilty of severely undermining public confidence in their own profession, to such a degree that it might take many years for Herbal Medicine to regain the excellent reputation that it enjoyed before the engagement in this misguided and disastrous adventure.

Excellent professional standards have, up to now, been built on the solid foundation of Voluntary Self-Regulation. This bedrock has sustained and increased the level of professional expertise within the established professional associations. VSR has also established a professional identity of sufficient integrity that in the past has encouraged a number of universities to offer degree courses on the subject of Herbal Medicine.

The recent strategy to "enhance" the professional status of Herbalists has implied a denigration of Herbal Medicine as potentially dangerous to the public; confidence in the reputation of the craft and the continued viability of the profession has been called into question.

The crisis in confidence invoked by such a campaign has been associated with a falling off of applications for university training in the subject. This lack of demand has led to several university courses ceasing to be financially viable, and several have been withdrawn.

The collapse of so many of the university courses focusing on the scientific biochemical approach to Herbal Medicine, isolated from its traditional holistic roots, has at least had the beneficial effect of directing the attention of those interested in studying the craft, back to the traditional academies.

The traditional use of herbs does not include the use of concentrated standardised extracts. These are now about to become subject to licensing under THMPD, to control the dangerous reputation with which they have now become accredited.

Although the prediction of future events is an occupation fraught with potential embarrassment, it is at present reasonable to entertain the perception that the "professionalisation" by adopting a model based primarily on reductionist science, may now be seen as a failed exercise in the evolution of the subject.

It is to be hoped, that in returning to its traditional roots, Traditional Herbal Medicine will be able to reclaim its excellent reputation for safety and efficacy, which it enjoyed before the current debacle. Some wholesale suppliers of herbs have become seduced by the perceived financial advantage of changing the natural into a semi-pharmaceutical product.

With the forthcoming introduction of THMPD, this has involved them in undertaking an extensive programme in order to obtain a manufacturers licence. This expense is in addition to that involved in actually licensing the individual manufactured products.

The forthcoming legislative landscape appears to be one in which the market in unlicensed manufactured products will not be able to exist, while the expense of licensing manufactured herbal products could potentially so increase the cost, as to make them no longer marketable on an economic scale.

This misdirected venture into reductionist biochemistry may prove to be an economic disaster for both the academic and biochemical industries. Those companies which have already invested heavily in preparation for a product that might now prove to be unmarketable, and may find themselves in economic straits.

While this is regrettable because of the negative impact it will have on the companies and their employees, it may yet least direct them to concentrate their business models on the supply of good quality medicinal herbs, to meet the requirements of traditional Herbalists and their patients.

***

Appendix I

A study of the Royal Charter, issued by King Henry VIII, gives rise to a number of interesting and relevant details.

Charter

Annis Tricesimo Quarto and Tricesimo Quinto.
Henry VIII Regis. Cap III.
An Act that persons, being no common Surgeons,
may administer outward medicines.

Where to the Parliament holden at Westminster in the third year of the King's most gracious Reign, amongst other things. For the avoiding of Sorceries, Witchcrafts, and other Inconveniences, it was enacted, that no person within the City of London, nor within seven miles of the same, should take upon him to exercise and occupy as Physician or Surgeon, except he be first examined, approved and admitted by the Bishop of London, and other, under and upon certain Pains and Penalties in the same Act mentioned: Sithence the making of which said Act the Company and Fellowship of Surgeons of London, minding only their own Lucres, and nothing the Profit or ease of the Diseased or Patient, have sued, troubled and vexed divers Honest Persons, as well as Men as Women whom God hath endued with the Knowledge of the Nature, Kind, and Operation of certain Herbs, Roots, and Waters, and the using and ministering of them to such as been pained with customable diseases, as Women's breasts being sore, a Pin and a Web in the eye Uncomes of Hands, Burnings, Scaldings, Sore

Mouths, the Stone, Strangury, Saucelim and Morphew, and such other like diseases: and yet the said Persons have not taken anything For their Pains or Cunning, But have ministered the same to poor People only for Neighbourhood and God's sake, and of Pity and Charity: and it is now well known that the Surgeons admitted will do no cure to any Person but where they shall be rewarded with a greater Sum or Reward than the Cure extendeth unto; For in any case they would minister their Cunning unto sore people unrewarded, there should not so many rot and perish to death For Lack of Help of Surgery as daily do; but the greatest part of Surgeons admitted being much more to be blamed than those persons of the said Craft of Surgeons have small Cunning yet they will take great Sums of Money, and do little therefore, and by reason thereof they do oftentimes impair and hurt their Patients, rather than do them good.

In consideration whereof, and For the Ease, Comfort, Succour, Help, Relief, and Health of the King's poor Subjects. Inhabitants of this Realm, now pained or diseased:

Be It Ordained, Established and Enacted

by Authority of the present Parliament, That at all Time From henceforth, it shall be lawful to every Person being the King's subject having knowledge and Experience of the Nature of Herbs, Roots, and Waters, or of the Operation of the same, by Speculation or Practice, within any part of the Realm of England, or within any other of the King's dominions, to practise, use, and minister in and to any outward Sore, Uncome Wound, Apostemations, outward Swellings or Disease, any Herb or Herbs, Ointments, Baths, Pultess, and Emplaisters, according to their Cunning, Experience, and Knowledge in any of the diseases, Sores, and Maladies beforesaid, and all others like to the same, or drinks For *the Stone, Strangury or Agues, without suit, vexation, trouble, penalty, or loss of their goods; the Forsaid Statute in the Forsaid Third Year of the King's most gracious Reign, or any other Act, Ordinance or Statutes to the contrary heretofore made in anywise, notwithstanding.*

Signed by

Henry VIII

The text of the Royal Charter demonstrates that:-

o   As early as the first half of the 16th century it was recognized that the conventional medical practitioners of the day were regulating their services on the basis of cost-effective reward to themselves, rather than consideration of the life or health of the patient. This mirrors the concerns expressed in the House of Commons select committee report, on the subject of the MHRA and the pharmaceutical companies.

o   The resolution to this situation lay in the hands of herbal practitioners.

o   As the Royal Charter referred to "every Person being the King's subject having knowledge and Experience of the Nature of Herbs, Roots, and Waters, or of the Operation of the same......" it clearly indicated the pre-existence of a culture and tradition of Herbal Medicine in this country. This remains particularly relevant in that the European Union has imposed upon itself a requirement and a duty to protect diversity of culture.

o   The Charter specifically refers to protecting the legal right of the herbalist to administer "drinks" as well as other forms of herbal medication. This specifically relates to the consumption of Herbal Medicine and not merely its external application.

o   The Royal Charter lays down legal definition of a practitioner of Herbal Medicine.

o   The Royal Charter has never been repealed.

Concern has been expressed in some quarters, that European law now takes precedence over laws enacted by national governments. This legal instrument however is a Royal Charter.

It is arguable that to overturn a Royal Charter would constitute overturning the Monarchy itself. To date, this point has not been challenged in the courts, and until such time as a ruling on this point of law has been established in the highest national or European court, any claim, by those seeking to deny the validity of this legal instrument, remains open to challenge.

Those seeking to have Statutory Regulation imposed upon Medical Herbalists, have claimed that this Royal Charter has been superseded by European Law and is no longer valid.

They have also claimed that there is no definition of an Herbal Medicine Practitioner in existence.

The Royal Charter demonstrates this to be untrue as it clearly provides a definition enshrined in Law.

***

Bibliography & Resources

Report to Ministers from the Department of Health Steering Group on the Statutory Regulation of: Practitioners of Acupuncture, Herbal Medicine, Traditional Chinese Medicine and Other Traditional Medicine Systems Practised in the UK May 2008

Extending Professional Regulation Working Group Interim Report: Protecting the public by ensuring that workforce standards are met, Dr Moira Livingston, Chair of the Working Group on Extending Professional Regulation 6th June 2008

A joint consultation on the Report to Ministers from the DH Steering Group on the Statutory Regulation of: Practitioners of Acupuncture, Herbal Medicine, Traditional Chinese Medicine and Other Traditional Medicine Systems Practised in the UK 1st July 2009

Extending Professional and Occupational Regulation The Report of the Working Group on Extending Professional Regulation

Prepared by the Extending Professional Regulation Working Group, 16th July 2009

The Law & Herbal Medicine - Regulation Facts and Fictions 10.11.2009.

House of Commons Health Committee Report from 2005, entitled 'The Influence of the Pharmaceutical Industry

House of Lords Select Committee on Science and Technology (Section 5.53)

Annis Tricesimo Quarto and Tricesimo Quinto. Henry VIII Regis. Cap III. An Act that persons, being no common Surgeons, may administer outward medicines.

WHO Traditional Med. Strategy 2002-2005

Herbal Medicine & the Law - A Critique

The Journal of Natural Medicine Volume V Issue 4 Winter/Spring 2001/2

Article 5.1 of Directive 2001/83/EC – COM(2008) 584 final (the) COMMUNICATION FROM THE COMMISSION TO THE COUNCIL AND THE EUROPEAN PARLIAMENT concerning the Report on 2a of Directive 2001/83/EC, as amended by Directive 2004/24/EC

Communication from the Commission to the Council and the European Parliament", dated 29/9/2008, concerning Directive 2001/83/EC as amended by Directive 2004/24/EC, on specific provisions applicable to traditional herbal medicinal products

Communication from the Commission to the European Parliament, the Council, the European Economic and Social Committee and the Committee of the Regions on a European agenda for culture in a globalizing world. Dated 14th May 2007

The RCHM's draft response to the Department of Health's Consultation Document.

URHP Response to Department of Health Consultation Document from the Unified Register of Herbal Practitioners 30/09/2009

URHP Response Postcard for members of the public.

Nexus June/July edition 1998

EHTPA Briefing paper and associated documentation dated 7.5.2008 to Mr Ben Bradshaw Minister of State for Health Services, previously available on the EHTPA website.

Correspondence between Gail Anderson of Human Resources, Department of Health, Social Services and Public Safety and Northern Ireland and the EHTPA, dated 15.1 .2009, previously available on the EHTPA website.

Correspondence between the HPC Chief Executive and Registrar and the (then) Secretary of State of Health dated 5.11.2008, previously available on the EHTPA website.

Copy of E-mail threat to URHP membership dated Tue, 14 Apr 2009 10:21 From: ELIZABETH LYDEN Subject: FW: [UK herbal list] 'Herbal Medicine' petition.
Extract from "Latest News" dated 15.1.2009 available on the EHTPA website.

Correspondence between Stephen Atkinson, Customer Service Centre, Department of Health and Robert Scott dated 3.11.2009.

Correspondence between Charlotte Urwin, Policy Officer, Policy & Standards department Health Professions Council and Robert Scott dated 9.12.2008.

Correspondence between Gail Anderson of Human Resources, Department of Health, Social Services and Public Safety and Northern Ireland and Robert Scott dated 15.12.2008.

Correspondence between Sharon Corner, European & It Specialist Legislation Team Workforce Directorate, Department Of Health and Robert Scott 26.6.2009.

Correspondence between Stephen Atkinson, Customer Service Centre, Department of Health on behalf of Andy Burnham, and Robert Scott dated 3.11.2009.

Correspondence between Robert Scott and Dr Moira Livingstone, chairperson WG on EPR dated 12.6.2009.

Correspondence between Robert Scott and Ben Bradshaw dated 8.12.2008. et al.

Report from BMJ Evidence Centre

Daily Mail article "8,000 killed in ten years by drugs intended to cure them," by Jenny Hope Medical Correspondent.

"1M a year are victims of NHS blunders or accidents," By Jenny Hope, Medical Correspondent Daily Mail

Why is NHS killing so many with drugs? By Daniel Martin Health Reporter (Daily Mail)

"Millefolium" the newsletter of Proline Botanicles

Timaeus, by Plato

Notes

Notes

Notes

Notes

www.ingramcontent.com/pod-product-compliance
Lightning Source LLC
Chambersburg PA
CBHW060629290526
45793CB00001B/203